Passion and Purpose:

Black Female Surgeons Volume 2

Stories and interviews to inspire and motivate young women to follow their dreams despite any obstacles.

By Dr. Praise Matemavi

Passion and Purpose: Black Female Surgeons

This is a work of non-fiction.

Text and Illustrations copyrighted

by Dr. Praise Matemavi ©2020910423

Library of Congress Control Number: 2020

All rights reserved. No part of this book may be reproduced, transmitted, or stored in an information retrieval system in any form or by any means, graphic, electronic, or mechanical without prior written permission from the author.

Printed in the United States of America

A 2 Z Press LLC

PO Box 582

Deleon Springs, FL 32130

bestlittleonlinebookstore.com

sizemore3630@aol.com

440-241-3126

ISBN: 978-1-946908-47-6

DEDICATION

To every child and woman
who has a dream beyond
what they can see.

Introduction
About the Book

Passion and Purpose: Black Female Surgeons is a collection of stories and interviews of black women surgeons from 27 countries representing the United States of America, the United Kingdom, Europe, South America, the Caribbean, and Africa. This book is Volume 2 and includes 33 of the 75 surgeons. These women were girls with visions who had the courage and fortitude to follow their dreams and embark on journeys that for most, no one who looked like them embarked on before. They set their sights on goals that were crystal clear in their minds even though at times no one else could see their vision. Surgical training is one of the most difficult of the training specialties in medicine and requires physical and mental stamina.

The contributors for this book overcame insurmountable odds. They are the definition of grit and resilience. They range in experience from intern to full professor. They are among the determined and fierce women featured in this book - The first African American female pediatric surgeon, the first female president of the Society of Black Academic Surgeons, the first African American Director of Member Services at the American College of Surgeons, the first female neurosurgeon in Uganda, the first female neurosurgeon in Rwanda, the first female urologist in Zambia, the first pediatric surgeon in Zambia, the only female breast cancer surgeon in Kenya, the first female cardio-thoracic surgeon in Nigeria and West Africa, the first female Zimbabwean orthopedic surgeon, and the first female pediatric and urological surgeon in Kenya. These and other phenomenal women share pearls of wisdom of how they achieved and thrive as women of color in a male-dominated field. All the surgical specialties are represented.

I was inspired to write this book when I finished my specialty training in multi-organ transplant and hepatobiliary (liver and gall bladder) surgery. As a child, I had the dream of becoming a doctor, but never had a frame of reference of a doctor that looked like me. This book has been a labor of love. I spent many nights and weekends contacting women via email and social media asking them if they would be part of this book. I remember wishing I had a book about women who looked like me doing what I wanted to do during my journey.

I read every book I could find about female surgeons. At the time, I only discovered two. I was motivated to collect stories about black female surgeons across the globe because we all have a unifying theme of grit, resilience, determination, perseverance, and experience of life in a way only those who look like us can relate to.

I hope all the brown-skinned girls everywhere in the world open this book and see women who look like them doing magnificent things in the field of surgery and become motivated to do whatever their hearts' desire. I hope girls and women are encouraged by these stories and interviews and will have the courage to take up space and flourish. This book is a celebration of those who have gone before us and the many men and women of different colors who have made it possible for us to reach our potential. We are certainly our ancestors' wildest dreams come true!

Dr. Praise Matemavi
Mississippi, USA

Table of Contents:

CHAPTER TWELVE: Obstetrics and Gynecologic Surgery (care of the pregnant patient and delivering babies, and surgery of female reproductive organs)

Dr. Keisha Bell Catchings (Practicing in Mississippi, USA)

Dr. Tosin Odunsi (Practicing in Washington State, USA)

Dr. Fatu Forna (Practicing in Georgia, USA)

Dr. Ruth Arumala (Practicing in Texas, USA)

CHAPTER THIRTEEN: Gynecologic Oncology (surgery for cancer of female reproductive organs – the ovaries and uterus)

Dr. Kemi Doll (Practicing in Washington State, USA)

Dr. Ebony Hoskins (Practicing in Washington D.C, USA)

CHAPTER FOURTEEN: Orthopedic Surgery (surgery of bones, ligaments, tendons, and muscles)

Dr. Samantha Z. Tross (Practicing in the UK)

Dr. Sonya Sloan (Practicing in Texas, USA)

Dr. Pamela Samoyo (Practicing in Zambia)

CHAPTER FIFTEEN: Cardio-thoracic Surgery (surgery of the heart and lungs)

Dr. Ogadinma Mgbajah (Practicing in Nigeria)

Dr. Lindiwe Sidali (Practicing in South Africa)

CHAPTER SIXTEEN: **Vascular Surgery (surgery of the blood vessels)**

Dr. Olamide Alabi (Practicing in Georgia, USA)

Fernanda Costa Sampaio Silva (Practicing in Brazil)

CHAPTER SEVENTEEN: **Ophthalmology (surgery of the eyes)**

Dr. Omofolasade Kosoko-Lasaki (Practicing in Nebraska, USA)

CHAPTER EIGHTEEN: **Otolaryngologic Surgery (surgery of the ears, nose, throat, head, and neck**

Dr. Gina Jefferson (Practicing in Mississippi, USA)

Dr. Barbara Grandison (Practicing in Montego Bay, Jamaica)

Dr. Tonia Farmer (Practicing in Ohio, USA)

CHAPTER NINETEEN: **Plastics and Reconstructive Surgery & Cosmetic Surgery (surgery for the reconstruction of tissue and skin and hair transplant)**

Dr. Metasebia Worku Abebe (Practicing in Addis Ababa, Ethiopia)

Dr. Sharone Jacobs (Practicing in Pennsylvania, USA)

Dr. Elizabeth Xoagus (Practicing in South Africa)

CHAPTER TWENTY: **Surgical Oncology (surgery of cancers in the abdomen, breast, skin, and soft tissue)**

Dr. Lori Wilson (Practicing in Washington D.C, USA)

CHAPTER TWENTY-ONE: **Oral and Maxillofacial Surgery (surgery of the mouth and face)**

Dr. Sandra Oyakhilome (Practicing in Cape Coast, Ghana)

CHAPTER TWENTY-TWO: **Surgeons in Training**

Dr. Josephine Kusano (Training in Zimbabwe)

Dr. Odinachi Moghalu Schulle (Training in the USA)

Dr. Weludo Ngwisanyi (Training in South Africa)

Dr. Ivy Godana (Training in the USA)

Dr. Amber Hardeman (Training in Louisiana, USA)

Dr. Rossana Chipalavela (Training in Angola)

Dr. Sharon Cheryl Bonya (Training in Malawi)

Dr. Nadege Fackche (Training in the USA)

Dr. Busisiwe Mlambo (Training in Zimbabwe)

Dr. Eman Abdel Elhassan (Training in Sudan)

CHAPTER TWENTY-THREE: **How I Became - My Story**

Dr. Praise Matemavi (Practicing in Mississippi)

CHAPTER TWELVE
Obstetrics and Gynecological Surgery

Obstetrician-gynecologists (OB/GYN) are physicians for the medical and surgical care of the female reproductive system and associated disorders. They serve as consultants to other physicians and as primary physicians for women.

There are also subspecialties in obstetrics and gynecology, requiring additional training: maternal-fetal medicine specialists are obstetricians/gynecologists who are prepared to care for, and to consult on, patients with high-risk pregnancies; and reproductive endocrinologists are capable of managing complex problems related to reproductive endocrinology and infertility, including aspects of assisted reproduction, such as in vitro fertilization (IVF).

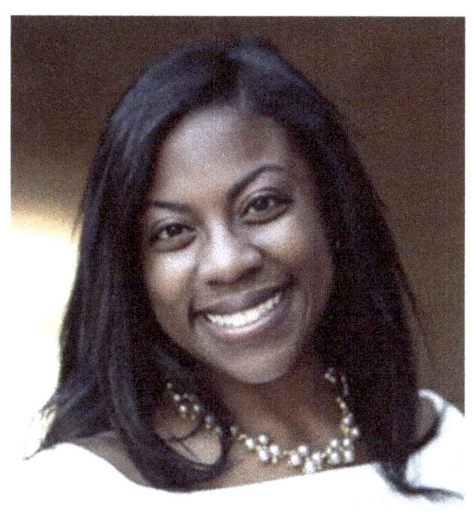

Dr. Keisha Bell Catchings

Dr. Keisha Bell Catchings is an assistant professor of

obstetrics and gynecology at the University of Mississippi Medical Center, Jackson, Mississippi. She received her Bachelor of Science degree in biology cum laude from Tougaloo College, Tougaloo, Mississippi, in 2005; her Master of Science degree in biomedical science in 2007; and a Master of Science degree in biomedical science in 2007. She earned her medical degree from the University of Mississippi Medical Center (UMMC) in Jackson, Mississippi.

She completed her internship and residency in obstetrics and gynecology at UMMC where she was chief resident her final year. After graduating from residency, she joined MomDoc, Inc. in Arizona where she practiced for a year.

As an active member of the American Congress of Obstetricians and Gynecologists, Dr. Bell Catchings has received numerous awards including the UMMC Department of Obstetrics and Gynecology Chief Resident Award, the Best Teaching Resident Award, and the Society for Maternal-Fetal Medicine Award for Excellence in Obstetrics. She has also received the Council on Resident Education in Obstetrics and Gynecology National Faculty Award for promoting high standards of residency education. Her research interests include the prevention of recurrent preterm birth in Mississippi.

This is Dr. Bell Catchings' story in her words.

I was born to Harvey Gales and Leesha Bell in February 1983. I lived with my Granny, Katherine Gales, for about five years when I was four or five years of age while my mom worked hard to make a better life for us. My granny is my heart.

I decided I wanted to be a physician when I was six years old. I was blessed to have parents, grandparents, aunts, and uncles who believed in my dream, even at that young age. They told me I could be whatever I wanted to be. My dream was nurtured from that time forward.

Through the years I participated in majorette dance as a Jackson Steperette, ballet, and piano. I returned to live with my mom at age nine. I was an honor student and was in the APAC (Academic and Performing Arts Complex) program from fourth grade through high school.

I decided I wanted to be an OB/GYN in the ninth grade after watching Dr. Catherine Hamlin, an OB/GYN, on the *Oprah Show*. She discussed the Hamlin Fistula Clinic she opened in Ethiopia to help women who developed vesicovaginal fistulas after childbirth. My friends were aware I wanted to become an OB/GYN physician and they, along with my family, encouraged and supported me. They even made future appointments with me.

I graduated from Murrah High School in May 2001 and began my undergraduate studies at Tougaloo College in August 2001, thankful for a full Presidential Scholarship. I never learned to study in high school because learning came easily to me. I scored well on the ACT having only read the small handout they provide when you sign up for the test.

College, however, was different. I struggled initially because I thought I could treat it the same as high school. I was wrong. By the end of my freshman year, my GPA was lower than what was required for the scholarship. I petitioned the Provost to allow me to attend summer school to attempt to improve my GPA. Though I did well in summer school, it was not enough to keep my scholarship. I was forced to take out loans to pay for the remainder of my education and I continued to struggle with learning to study. I earned a poor score on the MCAT when I took it during my junior year and applied to medical school my senior year.

I needed a letter written by a chairperson in the biological sciences department to apply to medical school. The chairperson did not know me but met with me to discuss my plans and goals. During this meeting, he told me he planned to write a letter stating he did not think I was ready for the rigors of medical school. I was devastated.

My granny was having problems with her lungs and was in the hospital preparing to undergo a lung biopsy when I discovered his intentions. I vividly remember going to the hospital to tell her what he said and how because of this, my dream would likely not come to fruition. She was livid and said a few choice words.

She underwent surgery later that day, aspirated and coded, but was revived with CPR. However, this was the beginning of a two-month hospital stay, including being in the intensive care unit. She was unaware of who we were while she was in the hospital, and we never had an opportunity to discuss it again.

Around Christmastime that year I prayed for God to give her at least a moment of clarity so I could talk to her and know that she knew who I was. Shortly after, I received a phone call early one morning to hurry to the hospital because she was awake. I jumped out of bed, threw on the first clothes I could find, and high-tailed it to the hospital. I walked in and she was watching television.

I said, "Hey, Granny!"

She said, "Hey," and continued to watch the television. I asked if she knew who I was and she said, "Yeah, Keisha. I don't know why y'all keep asking me these stupid questions."

I laughed out loud and cried. I still cherish that moment and thank God for allowing it to happen. The moment was fleeting because later that day she reverted to not knowing us. Things went downhill from then and on January 13, 2005, a family decision was made to make her a comfort care patient. She died that day surrounded by her children and me. I was her baby too. She loved me so much and I knew it. I was devastated that she left this earth knowing I would not be accepted into medical school and without seeing me graduate from college. It breaks my heart to this day!

I was not accepted into medical school but was offered a position in a post-baccalaureate program (post-bac) at UMMC, which I accepted. A post-bac program is reserved for students working toward a second bachelor's or master's degree or for students who want to strengthen their application to apply to a graduate or professional school like medical school or pharmacy school.

I completed the post-bac program, took the MCAT again,

and obtained a worse score than the first time. I graduated with my master's degree in May 2007, but I was not accepted into medical school. I was crushed. I remember telling my mom that maybe being a doctor was not in-the-cards for me and maybe I should dream a new dream. She encouraged me to not give up and that it would happen in God's time. I did not believe it.

On June 21, 2007, baby Jai was born to a close friend. She was struggling and I wanted to help, so baby Jai came to live with me when she was three days old. I had a new, beautiful baby. I never had a baby shower or any of the usual things when people have a baby. I figured it out as I went along.

Around August that year, I began working as a Regions bank teller. I applied to medical school for the third time and told myself it would be my last time. In December 2007 I received an email that I was accepted at UMMC. God blessed me just as I was about to give up. I realize now that the reason He did not allow me to be accepted before was because His plan was for me to raise Jai. If I was in the throes of medical school, I may not have felt as though I could raise her. He waited so He could bless me with the best gift I have ever received, my baby girl.

I began medical school in August 2008. Again, I struggled the first two years because even though I studied all day and all night, I had difficulty retaining the information. I struggled so much I missed earning a 75% score in physiology by 3/10ths of a point and was required to go to Georgetown in Washington, D.C., for six weeks between my first and second years to retake it.

I finished the course with a B. At the end of my second year, I saw a specialist, took a two-hour test, and was diagnosed with ADD (attention deficit disorder), the impulsive type.

I was provided with tools to help create a study plan to fit my needs. I performed averagely on my USMLE Step 1 board exam, but with the tools provided to help me study, I was able to increase my USMLE Step 2 board exam by more than 20 points. Throughout medical school, I balanced being a mom and being a medical student. People always ask how I did it, but this is difficult to answer because when you must do something, you just do it.

I learned to work hard and sacrifice from my mom. She did it because it was her only option. There were many times I brought my daughter to the hospital with me to study and she watched movies on her Ipad, ate snacks, and slept on her sleep mat on the floor in the classroom wing. I applied and interviewed for my OB/GYN residency during my fourth year of medical school and was matched with my first choice, the University of Mississippi Medical Center (UMMC).

I graduated from medical school in May 2012. My entire family was there wearing shirts with my name on them that read, "I'm with the doctor." They rang cowbells (since I was becoming Dr. Bell) as I walked across the stage. The love was palpable, and I knew they were so proud of me. We even made the cover of the university magazine because of it.

My residency training was difficult. There were many challenges and many struggles. There were times I thought I was not going to make it, yet I made it through. Residency graduation was such an amazing experience, the realization of a lifelong dream. I was blessed to receive my certificate of completion and the Chief Resident Award, the Best Resident Teacher Award (voted on by my fellow residents), and the Society for Maternal-Fetal Medicine Award for Excellence in Obstetrics.

I was so surprised because I still do not see myself as one of those people considered for awards. I do not know why this is, but I feel tremendously blessed that I was not only considered but I was chosen. I was overwhelmed with emotion because I felt that after all these years of hard work God was saying, "Well done."

I also had the opportunity to present the award I created in my daughter's name: The Jai Williams Board Award that pays for one rising senior resident's written boards each year. This is a resident starting their last year of training. I know what it is like to struggle financially in residency and wanted to give back. Since I did not have an opportunity to prepare a speech that night, I gave generalized thank yous. Here is the speech I want to share. The speech I wish I had said at graduation.

Thank you so much to everyone who is here in support of me tonight. There is no way that I could have made it through this if it were not for the people at my table tonight, as well as those who could not be here because of ticket constraints. To my mama, from whom I learned a fierce work ethic and the art of sacrifice, thank you for your love, support, your constant prayers; for always being there for me and Jai even when you are 2,000 miles away. Thank you for reminding me that I am still your baby girl when I say that it makes no sense that you are still having to help me at the age of 33. If I become half the woman you are, I will be blessed.

Thank you to my daddy who always told us, "Whatever you are in life, be the best at it. If you are a garbage man, be the best one." I have carried that with me throughout my life. To my grandma, thank you for ensuring I did not starve. To my aunt Yolanda and Uncle Aaron, thank you for your unwavering support, encouraging words and financial blessings throughout my journey. Thank you to my Aunt Jerry for your unwavering support, encouragement and for German chocolate cakes. To my brothers and sisters, I hope that I have set a great example for you; and that you know from watching my journey that anything is possible. To my cousins, thank you for supporting me and always letting me know how much I inspire you. To the man in my life, thank you for coming into my life at a time when I had determined that I would be alone for the rest of my life and for showing me that that was not the plan. Thank you for loving me through this and always letting me know how proud you are of me.

To my friends who could not be here, thank you for the calls, texts and Facebook posts of encouragement and for always believing in my dream. Thank you, also for continuing to invite me to events, even when you knew I would not be able to make it. That meant more to me than you know. To all the aforementioned, thank you for keeping me in your prayers. To my Thirsty Thursday crew, thank you for being such an important part of my life. I would not have made it through without those vent sessions.

To the little love of my life, my baby girl, thank you for being on this journey with me. When I have wanted to give up, I have looked at your sweet face and remembered that I am not just doing this for me. I pray that seeing me work so hard will inspire you to do the same in the future. I always worry about the damage residency has done to you with having to get up at 4 a.m. some mornings so that I could round and me missing important events at school because of work. I pray that instead of being scarred, you will be able to look back and say, "My mama set a great example for me." When you came into my life, I thought that I was being a blessing to you. Instead, you were a blessing to me. I love you more than words can say. Right now, you do not know what life is like outside of medical school and residency, as you were only one when we started. I am looking forward to showing you what real life is like. We are about to have some awesome experiences because of mama's hard work and the sacrifices we've both made.

Thank you to the attendings who have participated in my training; for teaching me the art of medicine and surgery. Thank you to Dr. Owens for being in my corner; for being a listening ear and a shoulder to cry on. Thank you for believing in me when I did not believe in myself and for that fantastic introduction that you did for me tonight.

To my co-residents, I am so glad to have been on this journey with you. Thank you for allowing me to be your chief resident and be our voice. It has been such an honor and a privilege. Rising third years, remember what it was like to be an intern and be kind to the incoming interns even when you are frustrated. Remember that it is possible to be tough on a person and show love at the same time. To the rising senior residents, remember that patience is a virtue and that those below you will be looking to you as an example. Be a good one. To all of you who will be here next year, be kind to one another and remember to talk to one another when you have a problem. To the #1 night team, you two are fantastic physicians and it has been such a pleasure to have been a part of your training. I know you will continue to make me proud. I love you and I will miss you all.

To the fantastic nurses and ancillary staff that I have had the opportunity to work with and get to know over the last four years: Thank you for being a part of my journey. Thank you for being on my team and working with me to provide the best patient care we can. Thank you for the encouragement, love, and support you have given me over the years. We have laughed, cried, and saved lives together. I love you all so much. You all mean more to me than you will ever know.

To my classmates, the class of 2016, it has been a privilege to share this journey with you. You all are fantastic physicians. The cities to which you are taking your talents will be all the better because you are providing care in them. I wish you the best.

To the patients that I have had the honor and privilege to care for, thank you for allowing me to be a part of some of the most wonderful and most heart-breaking parts of your life. Thank you for the many lessons that you have taught me, not only medical lessons but also life lessons.

Lastly, to My Lord and Savior: Thank you for every dark time, every valley, every "NO," every heartache and every ounce of sorrow because it makes me appreciate the tremendous blessings you have bestowed upon me even more. Looking back on my journey, I realize that ALL of it was necessary for me to become the woman and physician that I am today. You are so awesome, and You just continue to show this in my life daily. I thank you for my tests that have given me in my testimony. I thank you for every storm that has given me rainbows.

I have NO DOUBT that God is real. If He is not, I would not be who I am today. There are not many people who can say that a dream they have had since age six has come true. I pray that my granny and my granddaddy (who passed in November 2014) are sitting at the Lord's side and were able to see me graduate on Friday and know I finally made it. I hope I make them, as well as the rest of my family, friends, and supporters proud.

I want to leave you with this: I love butterflies. They are so beautiful and symbolize a new creation or new beginning. There is a story called the *Lesson of the Butterfly* about a man who saw a butterfly wriggling and writhing, struggling to get out of the cocoon. He decided to help by cutting the cocoon open and freeing her. However, the butterfly's wings were all wrinkled, dragging the ground, and she was never able to fly. It is the struggle that allows the butterfly to get her colors and fly. So, the struggle was necessary for her to be the beautiful, colorful, airborne butterfly God designed her to be.

Today, as I stand here looking at my beautiful wings (my accomplishments) and preparing to take off into the world as an attending physician, I am thankful to God for my struggle. I am thankful for those who stood on the side encouraging me and cheering me on as I fought my way out of the darkness and flew toward the light of my dream. The struggle was, indeed, necessary.

> You are enough!
> Keep your eye on the prize!
> Enjoy the journey!
> This too shall pass!
> This is where you are supposed to be.

"The greatest problem of human life is fear. It is fear that robs us of happiness. It is fear that causes us to settle for far less than we are capable of. It is fear that is the root cause of negative emotions, unhappiness and problems in human relationships." – Brian Tracy

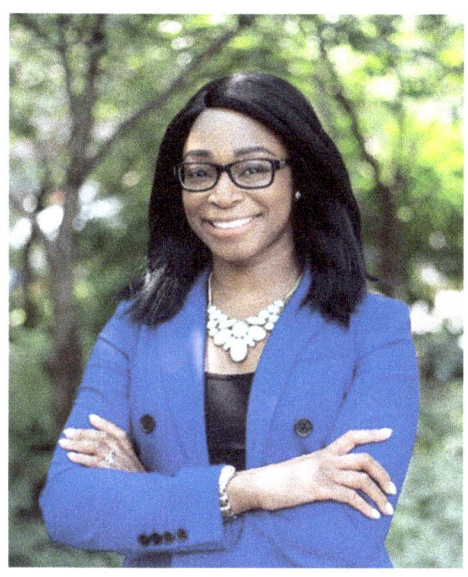

Dr. Tosin Odunsi

Dr. Tosin Odunsi is an obstetrics and gynecologist (OB/GYN) who has had a non-traditional path. After graduating in 2008 from Cornell University, Ithaca, New York, she started her master's education in Public Health (MPH) at Thomas Jefferson University, Philadelphia, Pennsylvania. She continued to medical school at Meharry Medical College, Nashville, Tennessee, and completed her MPH between her second and third year of medical school. She graduated from Meharry in 2014.

Sadly, Dr. Tosin became a young widow during her intern year of her OB/GYN residency in June 2015. This significant life experience has given her the courage to be transparent with her struggles and serve as a life motivator. She has since found love again and remarried. She has found beauty in her new normal. She is a coach to many and encourages people to live a full and intentional life.

Dr. Tosin is originally from Nigeria. Her family moved to

England when she was a child and to the United States when she was eight years old. From what she is told, she has wanted to be a doctor since she was three years old.

Her parents supported her but never forced her into medicine. Dr. Tosin's father is a gynecologic oncologist and guided and encouraged her along her journey. Seeing how much he loves his job encourages and inspires her. He still wakes up at 5 a.m. even though he does not necessarily have to and the passion he has for his job is always apparent.

Dr. Tosin's first memorable exposure to medicine was when she was in the seventh grade. She fractured her wrist and the orthopedic surgeon who cared for her inspired her to become a surgeon. How he fixed her problem with skill and gentleness was incredible and she wanted to be able to do the same for others.

She also volunteered at Roswell Park Cancer Center in Buffalo, New York, where her dad works. She had the opportunity to work with cancer patients, talking with them and passing out books. Later, Dr. Tosin also developed an interest in global health and wanted to incorporate this into her career.

When she began medical school, Dr. Tosin thought she wanted to be an orthopedic surgeon and she was the president of the orthopedic surgery club for two years. Then, during her third year in medical school, she rotated in obstetrics and gynecology. It was then she realized she wanted to do this instead of orthopedics. She felt she could have more impact and incorporate her MPH in this field because there are still problems with disproportionately higher maternal and fetal mortality rates among black patients in this country.

She likes this field because she can provide care for her patients throughout their entire lifecycle. She can take care of a lady during puberty, during her pregnancies, during menopause, and beyond. It is great to have the opportunity to care for multiple generations in the same family.

Dr. Tosin enjoys operating and this is probably the direction she is pursuing, moving away from obstetrics. She would like to focus her career on minimally invasive gynecology surgery. She loves fixing a problem and having instant gratification. She feels most comfortable when she is in the operating room and views surgery as an art. She is always learning from other surgeons and working on fine-tuning her style and technique to be more efficient.

Dr. Tosin would love to create a niche in fibroid and endometriosis management and treatment, both medical and surgical. This is because fibroid masses disproportionately affect African Americans and because of her personal struggle with endometriosis. It can take up to seven years to reach a diagnosis. She wants to advocate for women who look like her and are often overlooked.

Dr. Tosin has faced many challenges along her journey. She separated these challenges into academic and personal challenges. As for academic encounters, she has been a repeat test taker most of her medical journey. She took the MCAT (Medical College Admission Test) three times. She took both USMLE Steps 1 and Step 2 twice and had to take USMLE Step 3 four times!! Looking back, she says it took a lot of grit and tenacity to continue trying again despite the disappointment associated with failure.

Failing the USMLE Step 1 was the most devastating event for Dr. Tosin because there was so much hype about it being the exam that was going to determine her future career. When she received the results, she went through a deep depression she had never experienced before. She felt hopeless, useless, and worthless. To top it off, she only failed by two points.

She has a supportive family that encouraged her and reminded her of who she is and that an exam would not destroy her life. Dr. Tosin had to physically remove herself from Meharry where she was attending medical school. She needed time away. Her late husband and she were in a long-distance marriage at the time, and they had a home in Delaware. Her parents gave her the idea to take a year off to go home, retake the exam, and finish her MPH degree. This time away helped rebuild her confidence.

These are the times that test your faith. It is blind faith because it may not work out and you put in so much time and energy into your schooling. But this is what faith is. You must believe that even if your path ends up with your not becoming a physician, God will open another door.

For personal challenges, she lost her late husband Don the last week of her intern year. Her whole world came crashing down. Much of Dr. Tosin's identity was in becoming a physician and being Don's wife. When Don died, the bulk of her identity was gone. She faced the challenge of figuring out who she was during the remainder of her residency training.

Dr. Tosin walked away from God for almost a year because she was hurting so much. She could not even go to church. She was only 28 years old and devastated. It took time for her to find her way back to God. He was always there and waiting with open arms. She believes losing a spouse is one of the worst things that can happen to anyone, especially at an early age. If you can bounce back from that experience, a deep resilience is set for that person's life.

Another challenge Dr. Tosin faced was with impostor syndrome. Until she started her new job as an attending, she never felt she was smart enough or deserved to be a physician. She thinks the idea came about when she struggled with calculus in high school. She did not understand calculus, even with tutoring. This is when she began having feelings that she was not good enough or smart enough. These thoughts lingered until the end of her residency training. She was competent but not confident in herself. She needed time after residency to process everything and undo the years of negative thoughts.

Dr. Tosin has learned to speak life into her soul and spirit. She reminds herself she has been trained well and has everything within herself to succeed. She feels that for most new attending physicians the greatest fear is making a mistake that will result in the loss of a patient.

The reality is that physicians are human. No one is perfect but she knows that she will always do her best to care for patients the greatest way possible and call for help from more experienced surgeons when she needs help. She is at a hospital where she feels supported and respected. If she does not know something, she reads about it and finds answers. Plus, she seeks answers from those who have been practicing medicine longer than she.

One of Dr. Tosin's passions is mentorship. During her entire residency, she wore a mask and never presented her true self. She did not want to falsely come off as an angry black woman. She also did not talk about race. She had one black resident friend in another department who she felt comfortable discussing race-related issues with as they pertained to her training experience. It was nice to have someone who understood and helped her analyze frequent micro aggressions because she was experiencing the same issues.

Dr. Tosin regrets not advocating for herself but says this with caution because the truth is that people in power can retaliate if you call them out. It can be difficult when you see others who do not look like you have an easier time. So, for black girls, you must always be on your 'A' game. You must work three times as hard as everyone else to get half the recognition. You must not be on time, but early. You must be better than everyone else. She wishes she had someone who would have told her this when she started.

Dr. Tosin has been unofficially mentoring since college. She has mentored many women, but in March 2018 she started feeling alone and isolated because there were no physicians or residents who looked like her in her department.

She created The Mentorship Squad (TMS) which is a community of U.S.-based Black and Latinx women seeking mentorship along their journey to becoming U.S. physicians. The mission of TMS is to increase the percentage of Black and Latinx U.S. women physicians because these groups are markedly underrepresented. Dr. Tosin matches mentees with practicing physicians of the same demographic who are also passionate about mentorship.

Dr. Tosin feels sponsorship is the next level of mentoring,

someone going to bat for you. If someone does not match into a residency, their sponsor can advocate and make phone calls on their behalf. A sponsor must trust you and is more invested because sometimes they put their reputation on the line.

Now that Dr. Tosin has full control and autonomy of her life, she has more choices for how she spends her time. She is adamant about prioritizing her mental, emotional, physical, and spiritual wellness. Occasionally, she finds time to read for fun, and started reading *Grit* by Angela Duckworth. It is a great book about perseverance and determination. This is one way she finds balance.

Dr. Tosin read a disturbing statistic in the American Association of Medical Colleges in October 2019 stating 40% of women physicians switch to working part-time or leave medicine completely within six years of completing their residency training. Physician burnout is real, and by taking care of herself, she can hope to enjoy her career for a long time.

Two people Dr. Tosin would love to have dinner and talk with are her grandmother and her late husband Don. The last of her grandparents to die, her grandmother was a kind person and cared for everyone. Her house was always filled with people and was always giving. She was a praying woman and Dr. Tosin felt comforted by her faith. Her grandmother reminds her to be prayerful, grateful, and generous. Dr. Tosin's late husband, Don, died suddenly. She would want him to see where she is now. When they were courting, he promised her dad he would support her through her journey to becoming a physician and would make sure she achieved her goal. She wants him to see she made it to the finish line!!

If Dr. Tosin had to pick only one operation to do, she would pick a laparoscopic hysterectomy for simple postmenopausal bleeding. This is an operation to remove a uterus through a small incision using a long flexible scope. And, if she could choose the music in the operating room, she would pick Sade, but she would love to blast Afro beats. She is not brave enough to do so at this time. Who knows, maybe she will start.

Dr. Tosin's final words to all the young women dreaming dreams are, "You have everything within yourself to succeed. God has gifted you with the knowledge and skills and/or the ability to acquire the skills you need to become the best surgeon you can be. As with life, surgery is not about competing or comparing yourself to others. It is about learning, improving, and becoming the best version of yourself!"

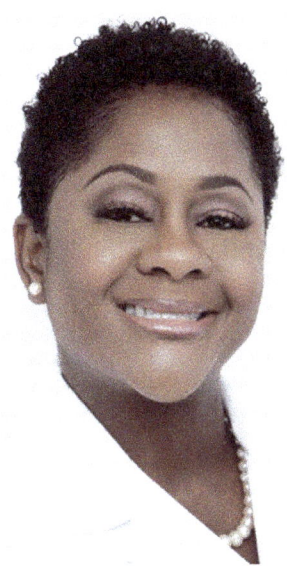

Dr. Fatu Forna

Dr. Fatu Forna earned her undergraduate degree from Florida A&M University, Tallahassee, Florida, and her public health degree from the University of North Carolina at Chapel Hill School of Public Health, Chapel Hill, North Carolina. She received her medical degree from Duke University School of Medicine, Durham, North Carolina, and completed her obstetrics and gynecology residency at Emory University School of Medicine, Atlanta, Georgia.

Dr. Forna served four years as a Medical Officer in the U.S. Public Health Service at the Centers for Disease Control and Prevention (CDC), Atlanta, Georgia, after completing her residency training. While at the CDC, she worked with HIV prevention programs in the United States and countries around the world.

She has also served as the Chief of the Department of Women's Services for Kaiser Permanente in Georgia, and as the Lead for Reproductive and Maternal Health at the World Health Organization in Sierra Leone.

Dr. Forna has authored numerous articles on sexually-transmitted-diseases (STDs), maternal and child health, and HIV prevention and care.

She is currently an obstetrician and gynecologist in practice in Atlanta, Georgia. Dr. Forna is married to a pediatrician and has four children.

She was born and grew up in Sierra Leone, Africa. Sierra Leone has always had one of the highest maternal and fetal mortality rates in the world. As a child, she grew up hearing stories about women and babies dying during childbirth. She heard things such as, "It was the first baby, she'll have another one." Even though she was young, this narrative influenced her to want to do something to change this. Dr. Forna wanted to be a doctor since she was six years old.

Her family always referred to Dr. Forna as a doctor and so this must have also imprinted in her mind that it was what she was supposed to do with her life. Her father had a library with many books, but she was mainly fascinated by medical books.

Dr. Forna clearly remembers the night before her 11th birthday. Her mother began to labor. She remembers the anguish she felt and how she was afraid for her mother to leave because so many women died in childbirth. Dr. Forna slipped into the car that took her mother to the hospital because she believed she could prevent her mother from dying if she was with her. Dr. Forna wanted to be the type of doctor that would keep mothers and babies safe, so obstetrics and gynecology was the only thing that made sense to her.

When she was 15 years old, the war in Sierra Leone was just beginning. Dr. Forna finished high school early because she skipped two grades. There were no medical schools in her country at that time. Since her mother knew she wanted to be a doctor and nothing else, her mother arranged for her to move to Tallahassee, Florida, to live with her sister, Dr. Forna's aunt. This way she would have an opportunity to study medicine. Dr. Forna discovered later that a medical school opened in her country the year before she left.

Dr. Forna arrived in Florida with one suitcase that contained all her belongings and two other suitcases with shoes, bags, and African clothes to sell. She received $1,500 from these sales. In her mind, $1,500 was not enough to live on and go to college, so she was determined to earn a scholarship. At 16 years old, she finished high school in Florida and her aunt used the $1,500 to pay for Dr. Forna's first semester college fees. Dr. Forna earned a scholarship because her GPA was 5.0 during her one year in high school.

By Sierra Leone standards, she was from an affluent family. Her parents had good-paying jobs. Her mother was a lawyer and her father was a politician. Regardless of their affluence, it was not enough to pay for her schooling in the States, so she needed to maintain good grades to earn and keep scholarships to help pay tuition.

Dr. Forna faced many understandable challenges adjusting to life in America as a teenager moving to a new country. Her uncle's job took them to Iowa where he was a professor at the University of Northern Iowa in Cedar Falls, Iowa. They also lived in Cedar Falls, which is not remarkably diverse.

It was difficult to come from Africa, where race is not an issue since most people are black, to a place where hardly anyone looks like you. Dr. Forna was not well-prepared for this adjustment. What she knew of America was what she saw on television, which is not realistic. She was able to make some friends, however, including a few foreign exchange students from other countries.

Dr. Forna's aunt and uncle did not like living in Iowa, so

they moved back to Tallahassee. She had two choices for schooling close to home with reasonable tuition, so Dr. Forna chose Florida A&M University. This is one of the best decisions she made.

At Florida A&M University, she found a great community; faculty members that cared about her growth and success and supported her. For her, having a community of support was critical because she was young. Dr. Forna joined the sorority Alpha Kappa Alpha Sorority Incorporated. She had a great experience during her undergraduate studies.

Though she was offered a full academic scholarship to the University of Florida in Gainesville, Florida, for medical school, she chose Duke University in North Carolina. This was because when interviewing for medical school, she met an amazing woman at Duke who was the dean of admissions, Dr. Brenda Armstrong.

Dr. Armstrong's mission was to diversify the school, so she invited Dr. Forna and other underrepresented minority students to Duke after their interviews for a second look over a weekend. Dr. Armstrong talked about her vision and showed Dr. Forna and the others how they would be supported throughout their studies. Another positive thing was they had a joint program with the University of North Carolina where Dr. Forna could earn a Master of Public Health concurrently and still graduate in four years with a combined MD/MPH degree.

Dr. Forna's Master's in Public Health is in maternal-child health and her research was in reduction of maternal mortality in Sub-Saharan Africa. She completed an internship at the World Health Organization (WHO) in Geneva, Switzerland. It was perfect for her. This experience opened doors for her to do exactly what she wanted to do, travel to African countries combating maternal and fetal mortality and working with the CDC.

When she completed her residency at Emory University Hospital in Atlanta, Georgia, it was a happy and positive experience. Most of her family was in Atlanta so she decided she wanted to be closer to them. The CDC is there and at the time, her interest was in doing a research fellowship.

When Dr. Forna interviewed for residency, she met a faculty member named Dr. Dennis Jamison who is now the chair of obstetrics and gynecology at Emory. During her residency, she worked at the CDC doing health research. During her interview, she told Dr. Jamison she wanted to do exactly what she was doing, working as an OB/GYN and doing research at the CDC. This was one of the reasons Dr. Forna wanted to train at that location. They had a multicultural patient base with many African patients. Whenever one came into the clinic, Dr. Forna's colleagues teased her that one of her African sisters was there to see her.

Dr. Forna's dream came true and after residency, she completed a two-year research fellowship at the CDC which allowed her to go to Malawi as part of her studies. She loved it so much at the CDC, she ended up staying for another two years. This allowed her to travel to other African nations including Kenya and Uganda. Like she said, it was a dream come true.

Being extremely fortunate, Dr. Forna and her husband recently worked in Sierra Leone for a couple of years. They moved their family home so they could spend time with her father because his health was failing. She was excited to be home and work on decreasing maternal and fetal mortality rates and is glad they made the move because her father died. She was able to spend his last years with him.

Her husband is a pediatrician and he also worked in Sierra Leone for one year, but it became difficult financially, so he moved back to the States. When she moved back, she accepted a position at Kaiser Permanente, where she is happy.

Dr. Forna's role is to help redesign their department to improve the quality of perinatal (all the care for a pregnant woman) care and decrease maternal morbidity and mortality. She is doing something similar as before, just in a different setting. She spends half her time doing clinical work and half her time concentrating on administrative duties. She has four children, one girl and three boys. The oldest is 14 years old and the youngest is seven years old.

Dr. Forna is a busy lady, but she is creative and talented and does some unique things. She is a writer and has puberty parties. Sometimes she feels like she is just existing because of the exhaustion from wearing so many hats. One thing that helps is realizing you can do it all, just not all at the same time. She gave herself permission to not be a superwoman. For example, she loved working at the CDC and loved traveling to different countries in Africa, but if you are breastfeeding and you have a baby, it is difficult and not practical. So, she had to give up the CDC because she wanted to be with her babies and breastfeed.

She knows that when they are older and if she still wants to do the job she did before, she can. Also, Dr. Forna has always had help raising her children. She had a village to support her. She may have moved out of Africa, but she never left the lifestyle where you have your family help raise your children.

At first, her grandmother lived with them to help care for the children, and at various times they had help from different relatives. Dr. Forna found ways that worked for her and her family. If she did not have time to clean the house, she hired a housekeeper. When she wanted African food for her husband, she catered it. Initially, she thought she could do everything, but it was not working. Figure out what works for you and your family, not what everyone else says is what you should be doing.

In terms of her writing, she authored a book for teenage girls called, *From Your Doctor to You: What Every Teenage Girl Should Know About Her Body, Sex, STDs, and Contraception*. This book gives teens the tools they need to protect their sexual and reproductive health.

Dr. Forna also adapted the book into a curriculum for pre-teens and teens and started hosting puberty parties. Growing up in Sierra Leone, no one talked to her or her peers about the changes one experiences as we get older, whether it is menstrual periods or sex. Her parents never discussed these things, so she had to figure things out on her own. Dr. Forna wanted to write a guide for girls. In fact, her daughter helped her with the book. As she wrote, she gave her daughter pages to proof-read.

For her puberty writing, Dr. Forna created PowerPoint slides and talked to her daughter about the changes she was experiencing. She is certain she helped her daughter understand her body and growing up more than most African parents do with their teenage girls. Dr. Forna decided to invite her daughter's friends and their moms. It became a party with food and cake, and everyone talked and Dr. Forna answered questions.

Initially, her daughter was horrified when Dr. Forna told her she wanted to have a puberty party for her and her friends, but Dr. Forna did it anyway and they all enjoyed it. Dr. Forna uploaded a short Facebook video clip and people started messaging her to host a puberty party for their children. The video has almost a million views. It has been incredible. Dr. Forna is terribly busy and realized she could not host the parties in person, so she created an immensely popular online course so parents all over the world can access the material.

Dr. Forna is also the author of a bestselling children's book series called *Puppy Princess Sheba*. She was motivated to write this series when she realized there are a limited number of books with black children in them. Since she and her family love to travel, she wanted to travel in the books. She wanted her children to see themselves in books and show them how beautiful Africa is. In these books, she chose several African countries and picked something special from each country. She was intentional in her choices.

For instance, for Nigeria, she chose a picture of Lagos with the skyscrapers to show children around the world that Lagos is as cosmopolitan as New York. For other countries, she chose unique animals to that country or the beautiful beaches there so the children could learn and enjoy reading. Dr. Forna also learned a great deal during her research; she was not aware that the largest church in the world is in Africa. She had so much fun creating the series. Dr. Forna feels writing was her calling, but as the oldest child, she felt a sense of responsibility to become a doctor, so she figured out how to combine writing with her medical career.

Dr. Forna feels her greatest accomplishment is realizing that life and your career are a journey and there are many milestones to achieve. At the end of the day, it is not about the milestones. It is not about the destination but enjoying the journey. It has taken her a while to figure this out. For example, when she moved back to Sierra Leone, she thought that was it, they were moving back home for good. It did not work out well for her family and she had to readjust that goal.

In addition to all she has accomplished, Dr. Forna has created a special foundation. a non-profit called the Mama Pikin Foundation. She and her husband are both from Sierra Leone and when they went home to help with health care, they noticed many women delivered their babies at home because they were ashamed to go to the clinic because they did not have anything to wrap their baby in.

This led to an even higher rate of maternal and fetal deaths because some of these women were birthing without experienced help. The beds in the rural clinics and hospitals were old with torn bed sheets. Dr. Forna and her Mama Pikin Foundation developed a delivery bucket.

Each bucket contains a sheet of plastic to provide a clean surface area for delivery, a Lappa (cloth) to wrap the baby, and soap. Each kit costs $7 and at the time this book was created, they have distributed more than 10,000 buckets. The buckets have been phenomenally successful in decreasing maternal and neonatal infections and provide an incentive for women to come to the clinics to deliver.

Dangerous home deliveries have been decreased substantially in the areas served by the six Mama-Pikin Foundation-supported clinics. The women who once delivered at home now come in to deliver with a midwife because they know they will receive a delivery bucket and also because the foundation pays for a motorcycle taxi to bring them to the clinic when they are in labor. It is not practical for a woman to walk a long distance when they are in labor, so transportation has been helpful.

Dr. Forna has three key persons that she would love to have dinner with and learn from. First is Barack Obama because she thinks he showed the world what is possible. When you have a goal and you aspire to something bigger than you could ever imagine, and you plan and you work towards it, it is possible. Michelle Obama is second on the list because she is a phenomenal woman, probably more amazing than her husband. She took a back seat while he ran the country and now, she is doing her own amazing things. Also, the president of Rwanda. She just loves him. Dr. Forna is not from Rwanda so there may be intricacies she may not understand that may make him unpopular among his constituents but for her, from the outside looking in, he is someone who was able to take a country that was poor post-war and bring the people together, allow them to heal, and transform the country into a stable society and economy. Rwanda is at a point where they are doing well. When she went to Rwanda, Dr. Forna was amazed at the way the country has transformed.and she would love to sit and talk with him and find out how he led his country to this level of reformation.

Dr. Forna added another person, her grandmother who helped raise her children. Her grandmother was not educated; her family was poor from a young age. Grandmother sold produce at the market to help support her family. When she was young, she married a Nigerian man who was a trader and had another family in Nigeria. He left for extended periods of time, so she created a business and put all six of her children through school. She valued education and knew that for her children to have a better life than she had, they needed to be educated. Grandmother's children did well. Dr. Forna's mother was a lawyer and her siblings also had great careers. For someone with little resources who could not read or write, Dr. Forna's grandmother worked hard and was determined to provide a better future for her children. Dr. Forna is grateful.

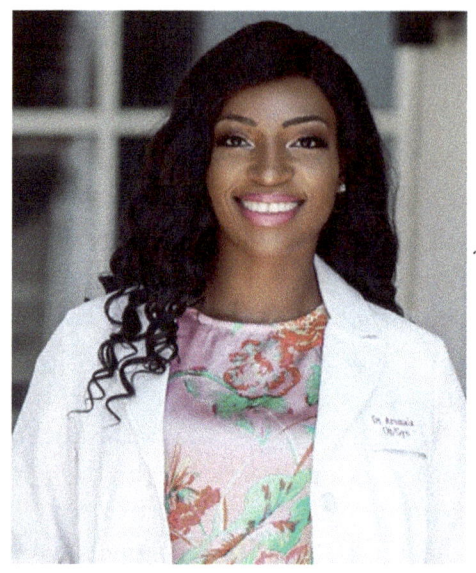

Dr. Ruth O. Arumala

Dr. Ruth O. Arumala is an obstetrician/gynecologist and women's health advocate with a solo practice in Mansfield, Texas. She obtained her Bachelor of Science in cellular and molecular biology/genetics at the University of Maryland, College Park, Maryland, as a Gemstones Scholar on a Banneker-Key full academic scholarship.

She also earned a Bachelor of Science in psychology from the University of Maryland, College Park, Maryland, and continued on to the Mercer University School of Medicine, Macon, Georgia, where she earned a Master of Public Health. She has a Health Administration Leadership Certificate from the University of North Carolina, Chapel Hill, North Carolina, and a Doctor of Osteopathic Medicine from Rowan University School of Osteopathic Medicine, Stratford, New Jersey.

Dr. Arumala completed her obstetrics and gynecology residency at Georgetown University, Washington, D.C., Medstar Washington Hospital Center in Washington, D.C. She received the following awards recently, her second year as an attending obstetrician and gynecologist: 2020 National Minority Quality Forum's 40 Under 40 Leaders in Minority Health; 2020 *Fort Worth Magazine* "Top Docs" Tarrant County; Ob-Gyn, 2020 Texas Super Doctors Rising Stars; and 2020 Women in Medicine's "Top OB/Gyn" Forth Worth. She is a member of the American College of Obstetrics & Gynecology (ACOG), American Association of Gynecologic Laparoscopists (AAGL), North American Menopause Society, and American Academy of Cosmetic Surgery (AACS).

Dr. Arumala offers comprehensive women's health services focusing on the medical and surgical management of pregnancy, fibroid masses, poly-cystic ovarian syndrome, infertility, sexual dysfunction, and menopause. She is passionate about empowering women to live a healthier, more fulfilling life through improving health literacy. She is a proud Nigerian-American raised in Salisbury, Maryland. She incorporates her myriad of experiences to offer the best and evidence-based care compassionately to her patients. In addition to patient care, Dr. Arumala is the hostess of the *Pretty in Pink Podcast: A Modern Guide to Women's Health and Wellness*. She embodies the *Pretty in Pink* woman as she exudes confidence through her voice, elegance through fashion, and strength through fitness.

One of her favorite things to do as a child was being dropped off at her mother's office after a long, stressful day at school. In her checkered school uniform and with her over-sized backpack, Dr. Arumala pranced down the hallway past all the other doctors' offices then made a swift right turn into her mother's office. Although her heart swelled with pride every time she saw her mother as a physician, one experience remains imprinted in her memory far more than the others.

Dr. Arumala's mother had a busy practice as a family physician in Port Harcourt, Nigeria. The number of people traveling in and out of her mother' office always impressed her. One specific day, a young man came searching for her mother. He spoke to the receptionist, or the unit clerk as she was called, asking to see her mother, Dr. Arumala. He did not have an appointment.

At the same time the polite woman explained that her mother had a full clinic schedule, her mother walked out of her office into the hallway with a patient. The man saw her and beamed with a wide smile. He rushed past the receptionist and started lavishly thanking her mother. She was too far away to hear each word but from what she could decipher, he was thanking her mother for caring for him when he was ill a couple of weeks prior.

He proceeded to describe a scenario that challenged the trajectory of Dr. Arumala's life. He thanked her mother for not only caring for him, but for also paying his clinic and hospital bill. Her mother had given him money for public transportation, to buy food, and fill his prescription. Her mother is unaware that this act of kindness formulated the foundation of how her daughter practices medicine today.

Dr. Arumala's road to medicine began in high school, where she excelled academically with minimal effort, particularly in science classes. Simultaneously, she was attracted to things that involved creating while using her hands. One of her side jobs in college was styling hair. She taught herself to braid, cornrow, twist locks, roller-set, and more. Dr. Arumala could look at an image and easily recreate it.

When she began medical school, she considered dermatology. In addition to the fact that the only physician she routinely saw was a dermatologist due to her persistently horrific acne, she also loved the cosmetic aspects of dermatology. As she continued in medical school, Dr. Arumala realized she would spend more time learning medicine than surgery if she chose dermatology as a career. She knew she was gifted surgically because she could recreate almost anything using her hands.

In the middle of her second year in medical school, six months before taking the USMLE Step 1 exam, her favorite person in the world, her brother, Samuel Arumala, died at 24 years of age. This devastating and life-changing event shook her to her core. It compelled her to truly investigate the path she would choose because she felt she needed to live out his legacy while living her life.

Still confused about her path, she took a year off from medical school to do research in dermatology and telemedicine. In addition to providing the necessary time for her to grieve without the additional stress of medical school, she secretly had time to reevaluate her path. During this year, she chose to pursue a career as an obstetrician/gynecologist.

OB/GYN, particularly gynecologic surgery, has created the avenue for her to impact the world. Her love for her patients transformed into women's health advocacy and a passion to prepare the next generation of OB/GYNs.

Dr. Arumala feels the challenges faced by black female gynecologists mirror that of black females in any field that is not traditionally ascribed to her. Her field is increasingly female, so her blackness seems more offensive than her being female. There is an expectation that all her conjectures, assertions, and instructions are shrouded in the image of the angry black female. In addition, her youth (or youthful melanated skin) does not always portend a peaceful transition in and out of the OR.

She was warned and adequately prepared by her mentors how to navigate her first year as a black female surgeon. One mentor advised Dr. Arumala to choose simple cases in the operating room to enable her to build rapport with the operating room (OR) staff in each new operating environment she encountered. Their trust in her skills came with time and she feels she had to prove herself more as a black female. Her mentor also encouraged her to practice professionally and consistently outside of the OR. This allowed Dr. Arumala to navigate the inevitable complications every surgeon encounters with more complex cases.

Most of her difficult days in training were due to false accusations, inaccurate blame, or plain hazing. (Yes! This is prevalent in medical training today.) Dr. Arumala shared her difficulties with her physician mother who also faced racism and sexism in her workplace. They shared these experiences. In addition, she worked out her stress and frustration at the gym.

Dr. Arumala has confidence. She feels confidence is deeply rooted in skill. The more you master your craft, the more comfortable you are taking over cases and pushing boundaries. But over-confidence is detrimental in most fields, and particularly so in surgery. Nevertheless, she still deals with impostor syndrome almost daily. As a woman of faith, she prays about her feelings of inadequacy and asks for the strength to be resilient and persevere. She also finds time to read her Bible to help her with life's challenges and keep close to God.

A typical day in the life of Dr. Arumala is anything but typical. She claims if you are a solo OB/GYN like she is, you know there are no typical days. On days she operates, she wakes between 3:30-4 a.m. She reviews pertinent information about patients including laboratory results and imaging for her cases. She also reviews the procedures and relevant anatomy. Then, she heads to the OR. After her cases, she sees patients in her office and/or rounds on her patients on labor and delivery, post-partum, the floor where the mothers who have delivered their babies are, or post-operative units.

On non-operating days, she wakes around 5 a.m. and does her morning ritual which includes prayer, reading her Bible, and working out. She heads to the office around 8:30 a.m. because her clinic appointments begin at 9 a.m. She usually sees patients in her office but may be called for a baby delivery or patient in the emergency department (ED), particularly when she is on call twice a week.

Dr. Arumala's schedule seems hectic but it is how she likes to live: a disruptive plan.

If she had to choose only one operation to do forever, it would be a total laparoscopic hysterectomy (removal of the ovaries and cervix through three to four small incisions using a scope to remove the organs) for issues ranging from abnormal bleeding to chronic pelvic pain. This major surgery can provide definitive treatment to many women while maintaining sexual function, urine and fecal continence, and ovarian function.

The procedural steps are almost always predictable because internal anatomy does not change. But as with any surgery, there may be things particular to the case that make the case complicated or interesting.

The best advice Dr. Arumala has ever received is to ALWAYS remain humble and hungry. Humility keeps her grounded. Hunger makes her grow.

The best advice Dr. Arumala can give is, "Take every opportunity to practice your craft. Do not take an easier route during training. Stay for the late, difficult cases. Anatomy is key. Study it often. Analyze your cases. Critically review your surgeries. What did you do well? What can you improve? Are there more efficient techniques? Better tools?"

And Dr. Arumala's final words to all young women are, "Dear black girl, we need you! The world needs you! Your community needs you! Through those almond-shaped brown eyes, you see the world with a unique perspective. Your strength and resilience are unmatched. Ignore the naysayers even if they look like you or share your gene pool because you are worthy of living your dream."

"Don't limit yourself. Many people limit themselves to what they think they can do. You can go as far as your mind lets you. What you believe, remember, you can achieve." – Mary Kay Ash

CHAPTER THIRTEEN
Gynecologic Oncology Surgery

A gynecology oncologist is an OB/GYN who has specialized training in cancers of the uterus, ovary, cervix, and vulva.

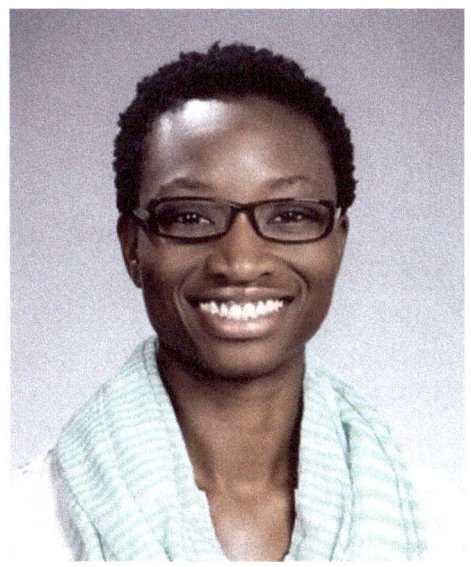

Dr. Kemi Doll

Dr. Kemi Doll is a gynecologic oncologist in the department of obstetrics and gynecology at the University of Washington in Seattle, Washington. She specializes in the surgical and medical treatment of uterine, ovarian, cervical, and vulvar cancers.

Dr. Doll earned her bachelor's degree at Duke University in Durham, North Carolina, and her medical degree at Columbia University in New York City. She traveled to Chicago, Illinois, to complete her residency in obstetrics and gynecology (OB/GYN) at Northwestern Memorial Hospital and returned to North

Carolina to complete her fellowship training in gynecologic oncology at the University of North Carolina (UNC) Hospitals.

Her clinical interests include surgery, chemotherapy, and hormonal therapy for gynecologic cancers and minimally invasive and robotic surgery. She is honored to be part of a patient's cancer care team and believes every patient deserves honesty, respect, and compassion. Dr. Doll brings these values with her to work every day and is energized by the unique relationship she has with each patient and their family.

Dr. Doll grew up in a city outside of Atlanta, Georgia. Her mother was a labor and delivery nurse, and this exposed her daughter to healthcare. She attended public school on the north side of Atlanta and grew up thinking, "I am going to school to be a doctor." Dr. Doll's mother is from Nigeria and instilled the importance of education in each of her children. Dr. Doll thought her options for a career were becoming a doctor, a lawyer, or an engineer. A doctor is what she liked. In college, she majored in biomedical engineering because she enjoyed biology but wanted to do something more interdisciplinary.

Dr. Doll attended Duke School of Engineering for her undergraduate studies. She received a quality education and learned a great deal, but the truth was she did not feel she had an enjoyable college experience. Her public school education made her feel poorly prepared for college. Because of this, she spent a great deal of time in the library. To be honest, she is not certain if it was that she was not prepared, or that she was intimidated. Due to many different factors, including a stressful home situation, she failed her sophomore year at Duke.

This was a difficult time but even after being academically suspended, she graduated as scheduled and was accepted into an Ivy League medical school, Columbia University in New York. The experience of going through failure and academic suspension and then needing to work extremely hard to stay on track to graduate on-time built tenacity and resilience in her.

Dr. Doll's medical school class was 25% underrepresented minorities and the Dean of Diversity was Dr. Hilda Hutchison who built a community of excellent students. All the students did well scholastically and had a great time together. Dr. Doll was the type of medical student who loved every rotation.

Initially, Dr. Doll was sure she would not pursue a career in OB/GYN. First, she rotated in general surgery and loved it. Then, she rotated in obstetrics and gynecology and, to her surprise, genuinely enjoyed it. In her third year in medical school, she chose to pursue a career in OB/GYN, a specialty she once thought she would never consider.

Dr. Doll feels navigating her path is her greatest accomplishment. There were many times she felt she was stepping out on her own and trusting herself and developed the courage to navigate her own life and career.

In addition to being a gynecology oncologist, she is also a researcher and spends 75% of her time doing research. One to two days a week she sees clinic patients and performs surgery. Dr. Doll dedicates one day to administrative work. She completes paperwork regarding her various research projects including writing scientific papers and applying for grants to support her research.

Gynecologic oncology is a specialty where she sees a mixture of different cases. For instance, Dr. Doll may have a patient with ovarian cancer that requires debulking surgery, surgery to remove all the tumor that can be seen by the naked eye. Or, she may have a patient with cancer that has spread to the bowels and may benefit from the removal of that section of bowel.

She also counsels patients and teaches them about their diseases and the best treatment options and schedules surgery when indicated. Some patients who see her are in remission, meaning that their cancer is not present at that time.

Sadly, she also sees patients that are at the end of their lives and she considers all palliative care options, making patients as comfortable as possible. Because Dr. Doll practices in a tertiary center, she receives many patient referrals from doctors at smaller hospitals with complicated diseases and provides a second opinion.

Dr. Doll's proudest moment was being accepted into medical school after her difficult college experience because it taught her she could succeed despite prior failures!! It looked impossible for her to be accepted into the medical school she was accepted to and yet she was accepted despite the odds. This became a tremendous motivator for her in her career and in life. It let her know that just because something looks impossible does not mean it is. There is never harm in trying.

Dr. Doll remembers the many challenges as a black female in training. She feels there is a double-edged sword of hyper-visibility. This means that everything you do is scrutinized. What she experienced was if you did well you were remembered because it was considered unusual for you to be in training at all and also because you are the only person who looks like you, so people remember. They remember you did well in that forceps delivery or gave a great morbidity and mortality (M&M) presentation.

On the other side of the double-edged sword is a very narrow margin for failure. Any little mistake you make is significantly amplified. People remember when you were late for a lecture, they remember when you did not deliver a great presentation in M&M, or that you missed a detail in sign out. (This is when healthcare providers hand off patients at the end of their shift to others taking over patient care.) Dr. Doll articulates these things well now that she has had time to reflect after training, but at the time she felt immense pressure to be perfect.

She saw a difference in what she perceived as relative freedom in her fellow residents or co-fellows. There were instances where after something happened, she said, "I could never do that." Whether it was not showing up to work, for a lecture, to M&M, or even in the types of emails that were sent to faculty and peers.

Despite all the challenges she faced, Dr. Doll did well and enjoyed the clinical work. She chose her residency program carefully and enjoyed what she was doing and where she was going. In fellowship, she focused on her clinical work and earning an advanced research degree.

The lessons Dr. Doll would like to share are, "In training, you must have a higher internal standard for yourself than anyone around you. You must learn early to set your own standard of excellence. It cannot be based on what everyone else is doing or what their expectations are because as black females we are either hold to 'too high' or 'too low' expectations. This is critical. I believe this was one of the things that helped me be where I am now. I had my own internal compass and knew exactly what I needed to do each step of my training. Sometimes the fire inside of us, our drive, can be misinterpreted by well-meaning mentors who want to protect us because they do not see things from our perspective and may worry that we are doing too much. But, if you have it in you girl, go for it. Go hard. Your standard must be high and your own. Also, deliberately cultivate a place of resilience outside your clinical or academic arena. A place where you remember what else you can do. Lean on your support people and have a place you can be 100% you and can recuperate. It takes a toll on everybody when you are this hyper-visible and you must have a place where you can relax and recuperate otherwise you will suffer from burnout early in your career. Take time out for self-care in your safe place where you can be your true self. And, lastly, you do not owe anyone your career, so it should be on your own terms. Trust yourself to know where you will thrive, whether this in residency or fellowship or your job as an attending."

After finishing medical school, Dr. Doll felt there was a great deal of outside input to her about where to apply for residency and this was the same for fellowship training. It was important for her to go where she felt she would grow as a professional.

She adds, "If you work hard and apply yourself, you can do anything, and doors will open for you. You are responsible for the quality of the career you will have. Do not allow others to make these choices for you."

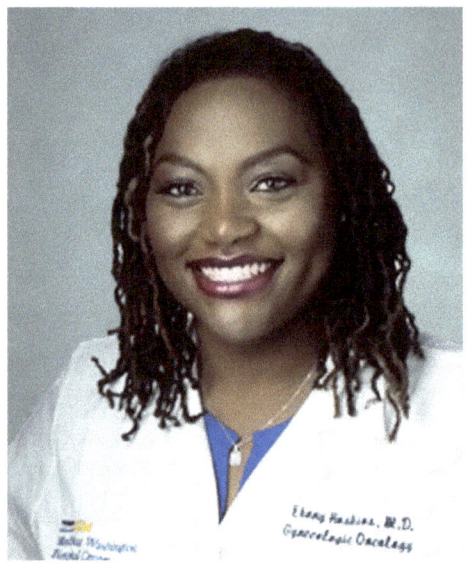

Dr. Ebony Hoskins

Dr. Ebony Hoskins is a board-certified gynecologic oncologist at MedStar Washington Hospital Center, Washington, D.C. She earned her medical degree at Wayne State University School of Medicine in her home state of Michigan. She developed excellent clinical skills during her obstetrics and gynecology residency at St. Joseph Mercy Hospital in Ann Arbor, Michigan, where she prepared for a clinical fellowship in gynecologic oncology at Magee Women's Hospital in Pittsburgh, Pennsylvania. She completed certified training in da Vinci robotic surgery techniques and qualifies patients for robotic surgery treatment of gynecologic malignancies (cancers). She has been practicing gynecologic oncology for nine years and continues refining her surgical skills.

Dr. Hoskins is a member of the Society of Gynecologic Oncology, the American Society of Clinical Oncology, and the American College of Obstetrics and Gynecology. She has been named a Washingtonian Top Doctor in 2016, 2017, and 2018 and has published various works including articles in peer-reviewed journals and abstracts.

She treats women with gynecological malignancies including endometrial, ovarian, vulvar, and cervical cancers. She sees women with complex gynecological surgical issues and considers minimally invasive surgical options for morbidly obese women.

Dr. Hoskins considers the use of robotic surgery because it offers patients many benefits including quicker recovery time, minimal hospital stays, and less postoperative pain compared to traditional open surgical techniques. She has completed more than 500 complex benign and malignant gynecologic surgeries using this robotic surgery technique. She also utilizes sentinel lymph node dissection for women diagnosed with endometrial cancer that may decrease surgical side effects associated with full lymph node dissection.

Her research interests include health disparity in women of African descent diagnosed with endometrial cancer and improving overall survival of women with ovarian cancer.

Dr. Hoskins grew up in Muskegon, Michigan. Growing up, she did not know anyone who was a doctor except the pediatrician she saw for check-ups and vaccines. She admired her pediatrician and in grade school, she decided she wanted to be a doctor. Dr. Hoskins remembers a time as a child she wanted to be a hairdresser, but her mother discouraged her from pursuing that career. After that, she never thought she could be anything other than a doctor.

A traditional student, Dr. Hoskins thought she was headed to a state school but was introduced to Xavier University in New Orleans, Louisiana. She loved the university and was accepted there for her undergraduate education. She attended medical school after finishing her bachelor's degree and followed the usual path, completing her residency and a research fellowship before completing her gynecology oncology fellowship.

As a third-year medical student, she was introduced to a program at Roswell Park in Buffalo, New York, where they were recruiting students to consider oncology. Dr. Hoskins completed a research project at Roswell Park, and this is how she was exposed to gynecology oncology surgery.

When she returned to complete her other rotations, she realized she did not love internal medicine and did not love obstetrics but enjoyed gynecological oncology. Dr. Hoskins was aware that to be accepted to an oncology fellowship she needed to be in a university-based program; preferably one that offered a gynecological oncology fellowship.

Dr. Hoskins did well in medical school despite not being at the top of her class. She earned an average score on her USMLE Step 1 board exam but did exceptionally well on her USMLE Step 2 board exam. When she applied for her Ob/GYN residency, she was invited to interview for 10 residency programs. Some of these programs were university-based while others were community-based programs. In the end, she matched with a community program but at the time, wished she matched into a university program.

Looking back, being accepted into the community-based program was one of the greatest blessings of her training journey. Dr. Hoskins had a great experience and did not suffer from burnout because she was in a smaller program. Unlike university programs that focus on research, which helps match doctors into gynecological oncology fellowships, her program did not. The first time she applied for an oncology fellowship, she was not accepted. Instead, she was accepted to the National Institute of Health (NIH) for a two-year research fellowship. This was instrumental in helping her secure a position for a gynecological oncology fellowship when she applied again two years later.

Dr. Hoskins' journey was relatively smooth from her undergraduate studies to her residency. It was not until she started her fellowship training that she began feeling unsupported and wondered if her skin color had something to do with this lack of support. She felt she was treated unfairly by some staff. Dr. Hoskins had to dig deep within herself to find the strength to overcome these challenges. She had to believe in herself and have confidence in her abilities as a clinician. Her goal was to finish fellowship, so she persevered and kept going because complaining does not help. She just put her head down and worked hard.

To build confidence, she read a great deal. This helped knowing she had the answers when asked questions. She made certain she was well-prepared for cases and performed well in the operating room to the best of her abilities.

Like all doctors, Dr. Hoskins has learned to deal with complications. She feels men and women process complications differently. She thinks men do not take complications as personally as women and are better able to compartmentalize. Men seem to better separate their emotions and are much more able to not take the complication personally.

Dr. Hoskins feels you must find a way to not let complications consume you. She does not expect perfection from herself because she knows no one is perfect except God. But she cannot relax until she has taken care of each patient and provided the best care she can. After complications occur, she wants to make certain the patient is better and is actively involved in her patient's care.

There are times when unexpected complications occur, and physicians need to know it is alright to seek therapy if these complications interfere with their ability to continue caring for patients. Sometimes there is no time to process these complications because many times when a complication occurs, the patient needs immediate care and you have other patients to care for as well.

Finding effective ways to deal with complications is imperative to prevent burnout and help your ability to care for the next patient confidently. You must remember all the great outcomes you have had and not focus on the negatives. You must separate the situation and remember that you are not a bad doctor and not let it paralyze you. Dr. Hoskins relies on God and the Bible for her strength and guidance, and she had a great co-fellow she frequently talked with. They supported each other.

On a lighter note, Dr. Hoskins' favorite surgery is a robotic hysterectomy with lymphadenectomy; taking out the uterus and the lymph nodes to remove cancer using small incisions and a robot. Patients do well, and it is an operation she enjoys doing.

She finds balance in life because her schedule is not as grueling as other disciplines and she enjoys reading as well. Currently, she is reading *The Purpose Driven Life: What on Earth Am I Here For?* by Rick Warren.

Some words of wisdom Dr. Hoskins shared are, "Apply to a program with mentorship because mentorship is important. Mentors help guide you and when you need an ally, you have one. Read. Reading develops confidence and when you are confident, others have confidence in you. When you do not know something, be honest about it. When there is a conflict, never try to resolve it alone. Make sure there is a third-party present. And, whatever you choose to do if your heart is in it, go for it!"

Dr. Hoskins' favorite quote is by author Leo F. Buscaglia, "The person who risks nothing, does nothing, has nothing, is nothing, and becomes nothing. He may avoid suffering and sorrow, but he simply cannot learn and feel and change and grow and love and live."

"A dream doesn't become reality through magic; it takes sweat, determination and hard work." – Colin Powell

CHAPTER FOURTEEN
Orthopedic Surgery

The scope of orthopedics includes the prevention, investigation, diagnosis, and treatment of disorders and injuries of the musculoskeletal system by nonsurgical and surgical methods. There are subspecialties as well, including: spine surgery, hand surgery, sports medicine, total joint replacement (hip and knee), pediatric orthopedics, foot and ankle, and orthopedic oncology.

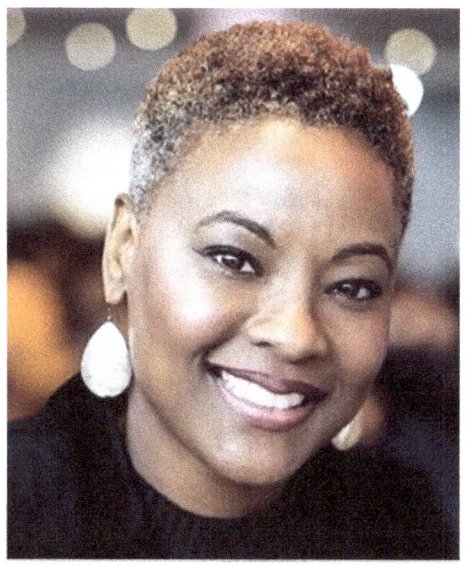

Miss Samantha Z. Tross

Miss Samantha Z. Tross is a consultant orthopedic surgeon in London specializing in conditions of the lower limb, specifically hip and knee preservation and replacement surgery. She is the first female consultant of Afro-Caribbean descent in the United Kingdom and one of 5% of the female orthopedic consultant surgeons practicing in the United Kingdom. She is a member of both the Royal College of Surgeons of England and Edinburgh.

Miss Tross earned her medical degree at University College London, England, before pursuing a career in surgery. She completed her surgical training at several London teaching hospitals including St. Georges, Guys, & St Thomas's and The Royal London. She also sought specialist training opportunities overseas at world-renowned centers in Toronto, Canada, and Sydney, Australia, where she gained additional experience in hip and knee surgery. She diagnoses and treats most orthopedic pathologies (bone diseases) and she utilizes minimally invasive surgical techniques whenever possible.

In addition to her clinical work, she is actively involved in medical education. She is an examiner for the Imperial College Medical School final examinations and an Associate Editor for the *Journal of Medical Case Reports*. She is an educational supervisor and mentors young surgeons, particularly female and ethnic minorities.

As a joint replacement surgeon in London, Miss Tross currently sees private patients at the BMI Clementine Churchill Hospital, BMI Syon clinic, BUPA Cromwell Hospital, and the Wellington Hospital. Her National Health Service (NHS) practice is at Ealing Hospital NHS Trust. NHS is the publicly funded healthcare system of the United Kingdom. The founding principles of the NHS are services should be comprehensive, universal, and free at the point of delivery.

Miss Tross has no idea what made her choose a career in medicine. She was seven years old when she announced she was going to be a surgeon when she grew up. Her mum was a nurse. Her grandmother and great aunt died at home. Miss Tross also had two friends that died when she was young – one from tetanus and the other in a traffic accident. Witnessing death at a young age had a huge impact on her. She was an avid reader and may have read something about medicine.

After being accepted to medical school Miss Tross knew early on she was going to be a surgeon. She chose orthopedics because the first female surgeon she ever saw was an orthopedic surgeon and she felt the orthopedic surgeons were the warmest and the friendliest. The specialty is nice because most surgery is done during daylight hours, and there is a diverse mixture of young, old, male, and female patients. Patients are generally in good health and recover quickly. This makes the results of her work quickly visible and appreciated. And, lastly, she has always been technically minded and enjoys working with her hands.

Miss Tross' greatest challenge has been overcoming self-doubt. When you are in an environment where there are few blacks and the system around you is filled with negative stereotypes, it is an uphill battle. She came to England from Guyana when she was 11 years old to go to boarding school. Her father's work kept her parents in Africa. Being away from her parents and culture made Miss Tross' journey difficult. The expectations others had for her were low because of the color of her skin. Her parents instilled self-confidence and belief in herself but without their presence, these were tested at times. Sexism is also an ongoing challenge. With more women entering the specialty, everyone is optimistic this will change with time.

Despite these challenges, Miss Tross has notable accomplishments. The first is becoming the first female orthopedic consultant in the United Kingdom of African-Caribbean descent. The second is being asked by one of her colleagues to perform knee replacement surgery for his mother, and another is being the first woman in Europe to perform robotic hip surgery.

A typical schedule for Miss Tross is starting her day attending a trauma meeting where the team discusses emergency admissions from the day before and plans care for their patients in the hospital.

Miss Tross is on duty one day a week and one in five weekends, but when she is not the admitting consultant on duty, she still attends the trauma meetings because she likes to have a consensus on treatment plans for the patients from all the team members. Then, she visits inpatients and evaluates their care and sees clinic patients with orthopedic concerns.

On her surgery days, she does not attend the trauma meeting. Miss Tross reviews pre-operative patients and then operates. She visits the patients after surgery to assess their status and order indicated care. She specializes in treating conditions of the hip and knee, so she performs knee arthroscopies where she evaluates and treats problems inside the knee with a small scope and camera. She also performs hip and knee replacement surgery. Lately, she has been doing robotic-assisted surgery.

Miss Tross is an educational supervisor for three surgical trainees (residents). This involves overseeing their career progression during the year they are assigned to her hospital. She meets with them throughout the day to catch-up on their progress. She also teaches medical students one day a week. She is also a faculty group tutor and oversees the educational needs of all the trainees in the orthopedic department during their four-month attachment.

With administrative duties, Miss Tross checks patient results, including labs and imaging tests. She replies to patient queries and reviews patient letters written by registrars (residents) before they are sent out. There is time during the week for personal reflection and keeping up to date with journals and courses. In addition to her NHS practice, she also works in private practice.

The best advice Miss Tross has received is, "There is no failure, only success and learning opportunities. Have a good support network and surround yourself with those on a similar path. Dream big!"

Miss Tross constantly searches for balance. This is a mindset and one you must work at she feels. Medicine tends to permeate all aspects of your life if you are not careful.

Her final words of encouragement are, "Believe in yourself. We spend a great deal of time worrying pointlessly. Believe that since you have been accepted to medical school, you are good enough to pursue any specialty. Give enough attention to your personal life. Plan to have your children if you so choose.

Get involved in research and innovation, discovering new methods to treat diseases or inventing new and improved medical equipment."

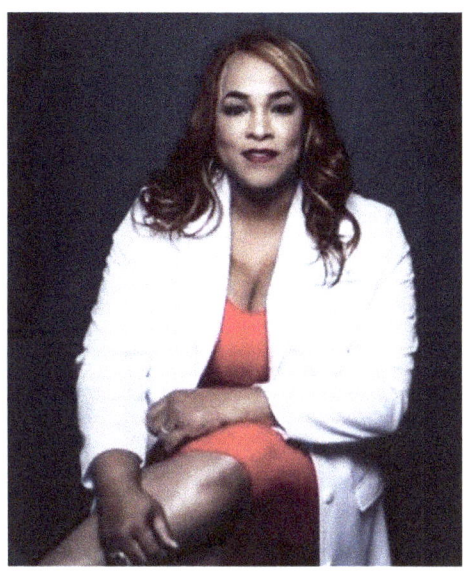

Dr. Sonya Sloan

Dr. Sonya Sloan earned her undergraduate degree in chemistry at Texas Tech University, Lubbock, Texas, and her medical doctor degree from the University of Texas Medical Branch (UTMB) at Galveston. After graduating from UTMB, Dr. Sloan accepted a residency position in surgery at Baylor College of Medicine, Houston, Texas. She was the first African American female surgical resident in the history of Baylor College of Medicine. She completed several published research projects in orthopedic sports medicine and was involved in a joint venture with NASA Johnson Space Center researching exercise equipment for the International Space Station Intermittent Resistance Exercise Device.

Dr. Sloan's commitment to impacting lives reaches far beyond the hospital walls and is evident by her work in her community and internationally. She has established two specifically purposed non-profit organizations, ME&WE, Inc. (Motivating & Empowering Women to Excel), collectively reaching more than 5,000 women daily. The other is SLOAN STEM+Arts. This is a faith-based educational diversity initiative whose sole purpose is to increase the number of minority students in STEM careers through early exposure and mentoring, impacting financial stability for generations to come. In 2015, along with the Luke Church, she initiated the philanthropic efforts for an international medical clinic with the New Missions Organization in Haiti that now serves a community of more than 100,000 men, women, and children.

She currently serves on the Board of Trustees for the Institute of Spirituality and Health. Dr. Sloan is a consultant, blogger, and speaker for DairyMax, a national partner to the NFL and Fuel Up to Play 60 initiative, helping youth improve proper daily nutrition. She has been an adjunct professor at Concordia University with a focus on health care administration. As a partner in RoweDocs telemedicine, she launched her Virtual OrthoDoc venture as one of the first of its kind in telehealth for orthopedics.

In 2016, Dr. Sloan was chosen as one of the TEDMED Front Line Scholars. Additionally, she has been listed as one of the Top 25 Women in Houston and has been featured in magazines and several national publications.

In February 2019, Dr. Sloan's first book, *The Rules of Medicine: A Medical Professionals Guide to Success*, became an Amazon #1 Best Seller in medical education and training. Her work in medicine, as well as being a respected motivational thought leader, has positioned her as a highly sought-after public figure and speaker for health awareness, entrepreneurial mentoring, leadership development, and spiritual enrichment.

A proud member of the Alpha Kappa Alpha Sorority, Inc., she is the First Lady of the Luke Church in Humble, Texas, where her husband, Dr. Timothy W. Sloan, is the senior pastor. She is the founder of God's Women Rock, a nontraditional, international annual awards concert that honors spiritual women from all walks of life making a difference for a greater good. Her three greatest rewards in her life are her children.

This is Dr. Sloan's story in her words.

I have learned to appreciate the saying, "If you want to hear God laugh, then make a plan." When it came to my aspirations to become a doctor and a surgeon, God's sense of humor was in overdrive. No one looked like me in residency. No one had a background like me. But perhaps that was my saving grace, because no one had a drive like me to make it and be the first African American female orthopedic surgeon at a top residency in the United States.

I did not plan for it, but each step led me to whom I am today. I did, however, pray for it. And I do believe that blessings will sometimes chase you down from behind. But heed my warning, be careful what you ask the Almighty for. You will never be able to script each phase of your life or career. I think this makes the intrigue and the desire that keeps us going.

As women, we are fighters and are perhaps the 'never say give up chicks with medical degrees,' that just keep going. We have a tenacity that will not allow us to stop and a craving for success that cannot be curved. And more than anything, we know that we know we have a date with destiny that will not let us quit until we have achieved what we set out to accomplish.

So, what does a woman, physician, and/or surgeon do with drive, tenacity, and a date with destiny? She succeeds and then learns to pay it forward; the term that has changed the world since the movie *Pay it Forward* came to the big screen in 2000. Random acts of kindness and philanthropic endeavors have increased exponentially just with the idea of a heroic gesture with nothing expected in return. You have probably been part of this movement as a giver or a recipient whether you realized it or not.

Considering the current atmosphere we live in today, *Women's Movement, #METoo, Black Lives Matter*, all encourage everyone to believe they owe someone something. Make no mistake, you did not get to where you are because of your grades and good looks alone. There is always someone standing in the background, in your shadows, and in the recesses of decision-making board rooms. These people advocate for you. Not always because you deserve it or ask for it. These people are the ones who know that sometimes it takes a gentle push or strong nudge to usher your success in a positive direction.

Think of every man and woman who spoke life into you, encouraged you, and/or prayed for you. Recall every face who helped you to be who you are today. And do not forget those who wanted to see you fail. I call them the nay-sayers. At times, they can and will teach you more than others do.

So, I did not give you the most helpful hints for huge success as a female who wants to go into orthopedics, but you already know it. Work harder than anyone. Play the game to win. You got this and I am here to remind you that you can do it. I did!

Lastly and most importantly, pay it forward. Do so because another young woman is looking to you for advice, support, mentorship, or just a hand up in a world where as women, we face unique challenges.

"Despite the persistent challenges faced by women in academic medicine, a growing number of us clearly are breaking down barriers. But in the presence of persistent conscious and unconscious bias and of stereotype threat, what is it that pushes amazing women physicians and scientists - what is it that pushed me - to forge ahead when roadblocks, incidental and purposeful, are put in our career paths? Tenacity and drive? Yes. Professionalism? Yes. Smarts? You bet. But I believe the key ingredient is resilience." – Julie Freischlag, MD

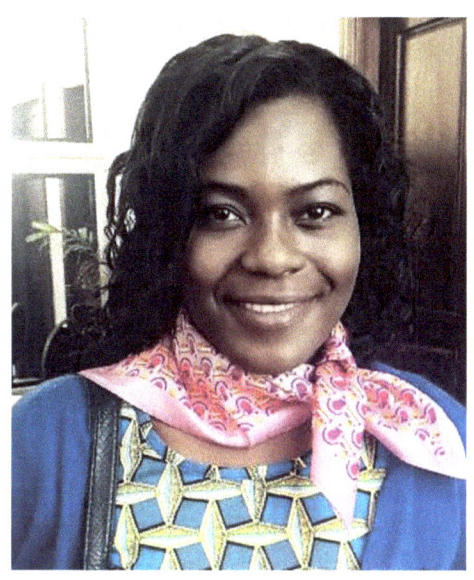

Dr. Pamela Samoyo

Dr. Pamela Samoyo is a specialist in orthopedics and trauma surgery. She earned her degree of doctor of medicine at the Ryazan State I. P. Pavlov Medical University, Russia (2010), degree of master of medicine in orthopedics and traumatology at the Kilimanjaro Christian Medical University College, Tanzania (2016). She completed an AO Alliance Foundation Trauma Fellowship (Kenya) and a COSECSA Oxford Orthopedic Link Pediatric Orthopedics Fellowship (Malawi).

She is an orthopedic surgery fellow of the College of Surgeons of East, Central and Southern Africa (COSECSA), Arusha, Tanzania. Currently, she is working as an orthopedic surgeon and serves as a pediatric orthopedic specialist at St. John Paul II Orthopedic Mission Hospital, Zambia. The hospital's main mission is conducting outreach programs and treatment for congenital orthopedic disorders free of charge to the needy and underserved community.

Dr. Samoyo is also involved in the treatment of adult trauma with interests in arthroplasty, surgical reconstruction or replacement of a joint, research, and teaching. She is a proud member of Women in Surgery Africa (WiSA) and has served as the treasurer for the organization since its launch in 2015. She advocates for gender equality in surgical training and leadership roles.

This is Dr. Samoyo's story in her words.

In high school, I enjoyed sports and participated in volleyball, tennis, softball, and other athletics. Growing up I wanted to train more aggressively in tennis and become a professional tennis player. Even though I considered becoming a tennis player, I was also passionate about and did well in science subjects, especially biology.

I balanced life between sports and school easily because I was passionate about both and had the support from my family that I could become anything in life without limits.

Because I loved science, I knew medicine was my field. This is a choice I have never regretted. Sports eventually faded from my life due to medical school demands, but nothing beats a good game of tennis.

My journey to becoming a doctor and an orthopedic surgeon has been difficult. After finishing A Level (advanced level) coursework in Zimbabwe (the equivalent of the first two years of college in the United States), I realized the country had one medical school that was not able to accommodate all interested students in the country. So, my family offered me an alternative to consider a different medical school at any university, provided the tuition fees were not excessive. I was accepted at Ryazan State I. P. Pavlov Medical University, Russia, in 2004 and my journey began.

The first few weeks after arriving in Russia were difficult. The racism I encountered on the street took time to become accustomed to. My brother, Dr. Brighton Samoyo, who was at the same university, encouraged me to keep focused on my goal of becoming a doctor no matter how difficult the studies and being away from home were.

After one month, I was able to brush-off the negativity

and never looked back. Learning the Russian language was helpful because the communication barriers where what made the first few months so difficult.

In class, the professors spoke English, but knowing Russian made my stay more enjoyable. I enjoyed the six years I was in Russia and spent time site seeing, and I even learned to ski. I graduated in 2010 with my degree in medicine.

After finishing medical school, I began a new life in Tanzania. I do not regret this choice. I asked my mother for assistance with travel costs to relocate to Tanzania where I was accepted for internship training. She was in shock! How could I relocate to a country where we had no close family or relatives and where I did not know the language? She feared for my safety. All the same, I made my choice and was determined to get there.

Tanzania welcomed me and I broadened my medical knowledge during my internship at Kilimanjaro Christian Medical Centre (KCMC) (2010-2011) but above all, it gave me a platform to experience the different specialties in medicine. I loved both pediatrics and orthopedic surgery and was torn trying to choose between the two. Then my mentor, Dr. John Burrell from Utah, USA, came along. Dr. Burrell traveled to KCMC yearly as a volunteer lecturer with Health Volunteers Overseas (HVO). Dr. Burrell gave me career guidance and he and his family made an offer for me to stay with them for one month in the United States to observe at Davis Hospital and Medical Center, Utah, where Dr. Burrell worked.

This one month of observation in the United States opened my mind and cemented my thoughts. I wanted to become an adult and pediatric orthopedic surgeon. I am grateful to Dr. Burrell, Dr. Lyman, and Dr. Bean who were all instrumental in my education and career choices.

In 2012, I began my four-year residency in orthopedic surgery at Kilimanjaro Christian Medical University College (KCMUCo), Tanzania. My residency at KCMUCo was difficult mainly because I did not receive a salary, bursary, or stipend. I only had family support to rely on.

There were many barriers and lost opportunities because I was a Zimbabwean national and was unable to benefit from applying for jobs and/or sponsored external rotation/short course opportunities. These opportunities were reserved for the local students.

Kilimanjaro Christian Medical Centre declined three consecutive job applications and could not facilitate my application for a pediatric orthopedic surgery rotation in the Netherlands because these positions are reserved for nationals. I understood this and needed to find a plan 'B' for finances and placement for my pediatric orthopedic surgery training.

The Internet became my best friend. I searched for scholarships online for short courses and worked writing online articles for money. In 2013, I had a breakthrough. The Cosecsa Oxford Orthopedic Link (COOL) program offered me a fully sponsored position in Malawi for training in pediatric orthopedic surgery. It was a six-month fellowship at Beit Cure International Hospital, Blantyre. The Department of Orthopedic Surgery at KCMC was opposed to my going to Malawi because this took me away from my residency for six months. Malawi was intended as a sandwich program with the pediatric orthopedic fellowship lasting only a short time in between my training in Tanzania. I am grateful Dr. Rogers Temu advocated for me to train in Malawi and because of him, the University (KCMUCo) allowed me to complete the fellowship.

The pediatric orthopedic fellowship at Beit Cure International Hospital, Malawi was a dream. I took advantage of all they taught me and was able to maximize my learning. I wanted to learn everything I could.

The best advice I have received is from my mother when she told me to think outside the box! Which box? There never is a box, which means there are no limits to what you can do.

Now, my days are all different, but if I pick one day's activities to share, I pick Tuesdays. Tuesday, at 8:00 a.m., we drive out with the team to a local compound or clinic for outreach. At the outreach, we screen children with orthopedic disorders and give them appointments to come to our hospital for further examination, imaging, physiotherapy, orthotics, and/or surgery. This usually takes until lunch time. Between 2-4 p.m., I see follow-up patients in the clinic for previously treated concerns.

My proudest moments are every time a child or patient with a previous disabling orthopedic condition returns to the clinic walking or smiling after surgical correction.

Balance can be difficult to find, but it is necessary. Balancing work, family, personal time, and rest avoids burnout. I try to find balance by daily prioritizing events like work, family and rest. It also helps to give everything you do your all, the first time and each time. I find this avoids unnecessary repeats. I also take time to read. Currently, I am reading *Born a Crime* by Trevor Noah.

I am grateful for all the Beit Cure Malawi staff. Between the years 2012-2016, I was fortunate to receive short-course training sponsorships that aided in advancing my career. I received sponsorships for the Cosecsa Oxford Orthopedic Link (COOL) program, the Institute for Global Orthopedics and Traumatology (IGOT) at the University of California, San Francisco, AO Alliance Foundation and SIGN. I am grateful for these. I graduated with a master's degree in Medicine in Orthopedic Surgery and traumatology in November 2016.

Currently in my career, I am completely in love with trauma surgery, pediatric orthopedic surgery, research, and teaching junior residents. At the same time, I felt I needed more hands-on experience, so I applied for a one-year trauma fellowship. The AO Alliance Foundation (AOAF) sponsored my one-year trauma fellowship in Kenya at Tenwek Hospital, Bomet and MOI Teaching Hospital, Eldoret. After completing my fellowship, I became a member of the College of Surgeons of East, Central and Southern Africa (COSECSA) after passing the exam in Maputo 2017.

Lessons I would like to share with the up-and-coming young female surgeons are build your confidence. Avoid apologizing unnecessarily. Do not allow others to make group decisions. Stop minimizing what you say and do not speak last. You are capable and your ideas are brilliant only if you tell the world. Learn to negotiate for better terms, for example, salary, flexible schedules, benefits, and more. Do not take criticism personally. Weigh criticism and make sure you understand what is being said, then use it to improve yourself or ignore it if it does not make sense.

The journey has been long. There have been many challenges. But, like a child in Africa who is brought up by the whole village, my career journey involved folks from all over the world. My career is a true definition of "I am because of who everyone was." I am grateful!

"All of us need a vision for our lives, and even as we work to achieve that vision, we must surrender to the power that is greater than we know. It's one of the defining principles of my life that I love to share: God can dream a bigger dream for you than you could ever dream for yourself."
– Oprah Winfrey

CHAPTER FIFTEEN
Cardio-thoracic Surgery

Cardio-thoracic surgeons operate on diseases affecting the chest, typically the heart and lungs but also the esophagus, diaphragm, and trachea. They operate on conditions that cannot be treated completely with medicine or interventional strategies. At times, surgery may be necessary for patients needing sampling of tissue from inside the chest to make a diagnosis, known as taking biopsy samples.

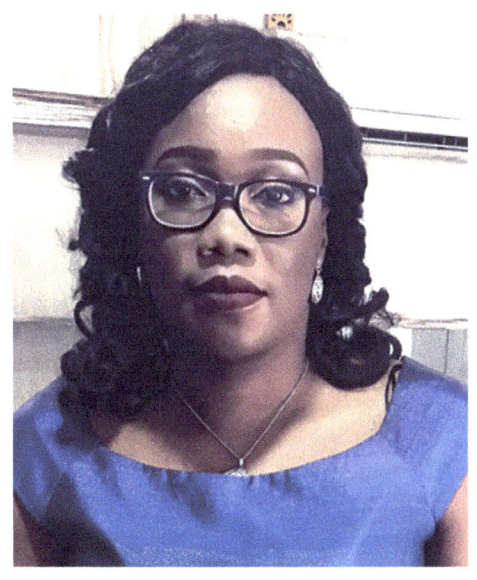

Dr. Ogadinma Mgbajah

Dr. Ogadinma Mgbajah is a consultant cardio-thoracic surgeon at the Tristate Cardiovascular Institute at the Babcock University Teaching Hospital Ilishan-Remo, Ogun State Nigeria, Africa. She is the first woman cardio-thoracic surgeon in West Africa.

She earned her medical degree (MBBS) at the University

of Ibadan in Nigeria. Following this, Dr. Mgbajah interned at the University College Hospital Ibadan. She completed her postgraduate surgical residency training in cardio-thoracic surgery and became a certified fellow of the West African College of Surgeons in 2016 and the first female cardio-thoracic surgeon in West Africa. Due to little availability of cardiac surgery in the country at the time, her residency training spread across India, the United Kingdom, and Ghana. In recognition of her achievements, she became the first recipient of the International travel fellowship award given by the Women in Thoracic Surgery (WTS) in collaboration with the American Association of Thoracic Surgery (AATS) in 2017, aimed at fostering global collaborations in cardio-thoracic surgery.

Dr. Mgbajah's clinical interests include both adult and pediatric cardio-thoracic care. She is involved in efforts to build a completely indigenous team for cardiac surgery at the Tristate Cardiovascular Institute which has successfully performed more than 400 cardiac surgical operations in both the adult and pediatric population in the past four years. This is no small accomplishment because most of the cardiac surgical work in Nigeria is still heavily dependent on charity mission work.

Her research interests include sustainable cardiac surgery in a resource-poor environment, heart failure management and heart transplant, mitral valve repair, adult congenital cardiac surgery, and thoracic oncology. Dr. Mgbajah is presently seeking to attract global collaborations with larger and more established cardiac centers around the world to help build a sustainable cardiac surgery program in Nigeria. She is passionate about creating more opportunities and creating an environment to train more female cardiac surgeons.

Dr. Mgbajah does not remember why she chose medicine. Her mum says as far back as when she was a child, she always said she wanted to be a doctor. While her siblings considered various career options, she always gave the same answer whenever prodded!

She definitely knows why she chose surgery! As morbid

as it sounds, Dr. Mgbajah looked forward to the cadaver sessions and, armed with a surgical blade, she dissected her heart out. No pun intended. Every other aspect of her pre-clinical studies seemed like a chore!

When she began her clinical rotations, her attraction to surgery became her passion. Dr. Mgbajah did not need to remember 25 possible causes of one ailment! With surgery, one or two possibilities for the causes of disease were enough!

Another consideration was she did not have to own patients for life. For example, if a heart valve needs replaced, she does so, and sends the patient on his or her jolly way. It is a practical specialty and she is a very practical person. So, it was love at first sight.

Dr. Mgbajah chose cardiac surgery because the heart made sense to her. All she had to do was draw a big box, divide it into four smaller boxes, put in gates (valves) and she was able to tell what happened if the gate refused to open or opened only slightly or if the gate flung wide open and refused to shut! She could tell what happens if there is an abnormal connection between the upper two or lower two boxes! Dr. Mgbajah was intrigued. She was hooked; it had to be cardiac surgery!

Dr. Mgbajah did not have challenges as a black surgeon because she trained in Nigeria where there are mostly blacks. But she did have numerous challenges as a female surgeon. Dr. Mgbajah had the support and backing of her family. It was an unofficial requirement for female residents, especially married ones like her. The question of having support always comes up in interviews! No one asked the male (married) colleagues if they had the support or the backing of their family!

She also had a few challenges with family. Most of the time, family does not have a full picture of what they are signing up for when they check the support box! Support in Nigerian culturally means being a wife, mother, and managing a home excellently (making meals, keeping the home) while being an excellent resident. The home cannot suffer because you have ambition! And culture requires you have a home (children and all) at a certain age. Dr. Mgbajah had three boys while training as a cardio-thoracic surgeon. It was an uphill task because she traveled to various countries to learn the skills she needed because cardio-thoracic surgery is still in its infant stages in Nigeria. Wherever she went, her family went.

It is bad enough Dr. Mgbajah dared to dream of becoming a surgeon as a female. Pediatric surgery was understandable, but she took her choices a notch higher and wanted to become a cardio-thoracic surgeon. Dr. Mgbajah dared to walk the paths trod exclusively by men! She endured the snide remarks, "Go and take care of your home!" "Can you saw open the sternum?" "Can you wire the sternum?"

Whenever she introduced herself as a resident in cardio-thoracic surgery, the reactions were predictable. No one paid attention! "She will change her mind." "How would she cope? Not going home for days?" were just a few of the common comments. Dr. Mgbajah was even rotated out of cases to favor male residents visiting from other hospitals, but she made her trainers and consultants believers, one after another!

Dr. Mgbajah was not always confident. She had timid moments and her, "I can't do this anymore" moments. She had her self-doubt moments and still does. A bit of self-doubt helps one grow. Dr. Mgbajah had moments when everything seemed to be going south, but thankfully, these times were transient, and confidence triumphed.

She feels there are many ways to build confidence. One way is knowledge. Dr. Mgbajah sought knowledge. She researched, read books and journals, and attended conferences. She made certain she knew her material! There is a level of confidence that comes with knowledge.

Another way to build confidence is practice. Dr. Mgbajah did things repetitively! She practiced suturing on cut pieces of foam! Those hand knots – she tied them over and over, frustrated at first and over time, it became second nature.

A third way to build confidence is mentors. The role of mentors cannot be overemphasized. In her case, it was friends.

Dr. Mgbajah had two girlfriends training in general surgery and urology at the same time. They bounced ideas off each other, encouraged each other, picked up what was left of each other's confidence from time to time, and polished it till it shone!

A typical day in her part of the world as a cardio-thoracic surgeon in practice is anything but typical. They do not have work hours. Days easily roll into nights and nights into days, as they wear so many hats – surgeons, intensivists, respiratory therapists, and more. Dr. Mgbajah and her team rest when a surgical patient is discharged and there is often a break when there are no patients to operate on! Cardio-thoracic surgical practice in the most active center in a third-world country is an entirely different book of experiences.

Dr. Mgbajah's proudest moment was the day she received her degree and her award as the first female cardio-thoracic surgeon in Nigeria and West Africa, all with her husband and three sons by her side. This day she felt as though she had truly shattered the glass ceiling.

She gives heartfelt thanks to her husband, her sons and family, Mr. Bode Falase and Dr. Michael Sanusi (her primary trainers), and Dr. AGK Gokhale, Dr. Lauren Kane, Dr. Emily Farkas, Dr. O. C Nzewi (her secondary trainers). Seven years and three continents later, she became the first and only female cardio-thoracic surgeon in Nigeria and West Africa.

The best advice Dr. Mgbajah received is, *"You are responsible for how you turn out! Never delegate this all-important responsibility to any person, circumstance, or environment."* Her favorite quotes in residency were: "Every storm runs out of rain." (Maya Angelou) and *"And it came to pass." (The Bible).*

Dr. Mgbajah would like to share a few truths she has come to embrace in her journey, "Pace yourself. Run your race! Do not try to achieve another person's goal. Small victories add up and are easier to achieve! So, instead of wearing yourself out aiming for a huge dramatic win, aim for one small victory at a time. Trust me, the feeling is the same. Do not lose focus. Eventually, it will all add up. You are training to become a SURGEON, not a female surgeon! Notice our male colleagues do not refer to themselves as male surgeons. This is because the profession is surgery, your gender is your business! Don't accept lower standards, fewer calls, or less work because you are a female surgeon. Do not let anyone ask you if you need to scrub-out or if you want to rest a bit because you are a female surgeon. You are a surgeon, period! Show up. Put in the work and show out. Make certain your vision is clear and your motives are correct. Gather all the necessary information to make informed decisions, including options for places to train. When you have adequately counted the costs, get up and get it done. Pace yourself. Run your race. Set goals. Do not try to achieve goals set by others. It is a marathon and you've got this!"

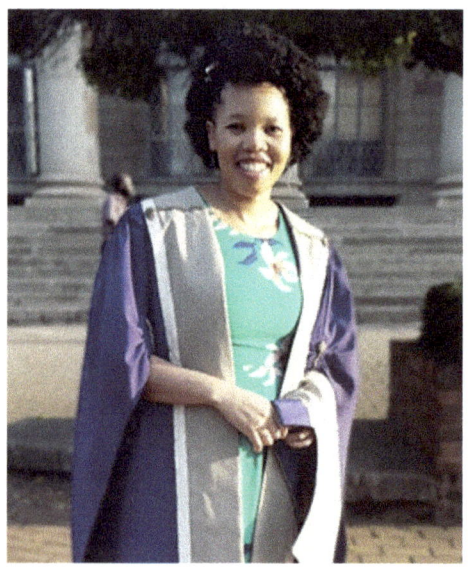

Dr. Lindiwe Sidali

Dr. Lindiwe Sidali is a cardio-thoracic surgeon at Inkosi Albert Luthuli Central Hospital, in Durban, South Africa. She received her medical degree from Facultad de Ciencias Medicas Sancti Spiritus, Cuba, and her training in cardio-thoracic surgery at Inkosi Albert Luthuli Central Hospital, Durban, Kwa-Zulu Natal.

Dr. Sidali's journey began a long time before she became an accomplished cardio-thoracic surgeon. She was born in a large family of eight in a small town called Dutywa, in the Eastern Cape, South Africa. Her father worked in the Wonderkop mine in Rusternburg, North West, so she lived between the two provinces.

She attended Rakgatla High School in Wonderkop and earned a bursary (scholarship) from the North West Department of Health to study medicine in Cuba. Dr. Sidali's parents were true feminists, so to speak. All the children in her family were treated equally in a culture that tends to have defined gender roles. Whether you were a girl or a boy, you were expected to cook, clean, and herd cattle and perform to the best of your abilities in school. Her parents taught Dr. Sidali and her siblings the value of hard work.

When she was in high school, Dr. Sidali volunteered at the Wonderkop clinic. The nurses there were wonderful and encouraged her to pursue medicine. Her family and teachers were also supportive and encouraging. While volunteering at the clinic, Dr. Sidali learned of the Southern African-Cuban scholarship to study medicine.

She applied and was accepted. She was interested in medicine because she has always wanted to serve her people and give back, not only by being a doctor but also by serving as a positive role model for every African child. Dr. Sidali wants to show them they can achieve anything they desire.

As for cardio-thoracic surgery, it happened by chance. During her rotations in medical school, she was interested in surgical disciplines but did not know which one to pursue. While rotating in general surgery, she was also a house officer completing her community service. In South Africa, physicians are required to do community service before they can complete official residency training. One day, a patient came to the hospital with a stab wound to the heart. The patient was taken to the operating room and, after experiencing a heart beating in her hands, she knew she wanted to become a cardio-thoracic surgeon.

Dr. Sidali does not think of her journey as a sacrifice. To her, it was time well-spent as she focused on her studies and advancing in her career. She has been fortunate to have many people supporting her and cheering her on along the way. She is grateful that her family has always been the cheerleaders of her life and her teachers too, the ones who expected the best from her.

She is grateful for her friends who were there for her through it all and everyone who saw potential in her and gave her a chance. From the Department of Health, North West, and to the Cuban community for their warm welcome and the knowledge they shared in medicine, they also taught Dr. Sidali to be proud of who she is and where she comes from.

She is also thankful to her mentors for the guidance and advice they generously gave, for believing in her and supporting her throughout her journey. She thanks the KZN Department of Health for its support. And, finally, she is grateful for the professors who taught her the art of surgery.

When she was asked what barriers she feels women face to achieve success in male-dominated fields, Dr. Sidali shared, "It is difficult to answer this question without sparking debate in other areas, but I suppose it is the same reason we still have not had a female president. These same barriers need to be broken. It is only when people see that one female can do it that they can give a chance to other females. It is uncharted territory for females, particularly African females because they are hardly ever given a chance. In my opinion, when women are given the same position as men, they are tested to the point of failure. This is where all intuitive direction points one to believe they cannot do it. So, the odds for African women are systematically, probably unintentionally, designed to drive us to not fight for more or to quit."

Dr. Sidali feels there is an increase in the number of

female doctors in surgical disciplines overall. These disciplines have been famously known as the boy's club. However, African females have been given the least opportunities compared to their counterparts. They need opportunities and exposure. The most important thing that needs to change the future for all African children is the eradication of poverty. One way to do this is through education. This is how to truly liberate a person. But education requires money, which is the reason education needs to be free for those from disadvantaged backgrounds. There also to be more positive role models for young women. African girls need to see a girl who looks like them achieving success. This way they can see it can be done.

Dr. Sidali asserts her present position is just the beginning of a new dawn. She is excited to hit the ground running and sharpen her skills even more and teach and transfer her skills to the next generation of surgeons. She plans to pursue congenital cardiac surgery, a sub-specialty/super specialty in cardio-thoracic surgery dealing with structural problems of the heart present from birth. These structural defects range from a small hole between the heart chambers to complex abnormalities such as an abnormal spatial arrangement of the great blood vessels.

Dr. Sidali describes herself as aware. She is aware of herself, who she is and what she stands for, making it easier for others to be aware of her. She also describes herself as feminist, decisive, a dreamer, and dauntless.

She shares how she writes romantic fiction stories, but only for her friends, as she writes under a pseudo name. She intends to share her writing with the world someday, but no one will ever know it is her. Now that she has finished her exams, besides working hard, she is planning to practice more of her hobbies.

Dr. Sidali's final words are, "Everything in life is possible. Dream but create a plan of action in achieving those goals. Do not follow other people's paths. Create a new one for yourself and others."

CHAPTER SIXTEEN
Vascular Surgery

Vascular surgery is a surgical subspecialty in which diseases of the vascular system, or arteries, veins, and lymphatic circulation, are managed by medical therapy, minimally-invasive catheter procedures, and surgical reconstruction. The vascular surgeon is trained in the diagnosis and management of diseases affecting all parts of the vascular system excluding the coronaries and intracranial vasculature.

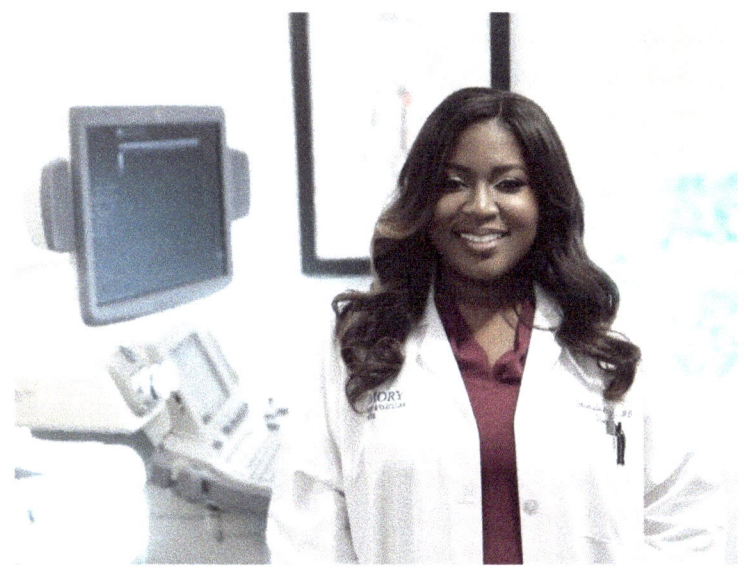

Dr. Olamide Alabi

Dr. Olamide Alabi is a vascular surgeon at Emory University Hospital in Atlanta, Georgia. She received her medical degree from the University of Nebraska, College of Medicine, Omaha, Nebraska, trained in general surgery at Loma Linda University Medical Center in Loma Linda, California, and completed her fellowship in vascular surgery at Oregon Health and Science University, Portland, Oregon.

This is Dr. Alabi's story in her words.

When I was earning my undergraduate degree at the University of Nebraska, Omaha, I was interested in finding a scholarship for students who were underrepresented minorities and from low-income families as well as first-generation college students.

At that time, I was not interested in medicine, but I did need a scholarship. As part of the program, we were required to go to the hospital, where I became interested in medicine. I stayed in the program and attended the medical school associated with the program, the University of Nebraska Medical School. Initially, I considered psychiatry, but felt this was depressing because I did not see tangible results.

During my first year in medical school, I accompanied a few primary-care physicians on a medical mission trip to Mexico. It was then that I realized I did not feel fulfilled treating medical conditions and returning to my life in the United States knowing there was no one in Mexico to follow up with the patients we cared for.

And, in my second year in medical school, I accompanied another team on a surgical mission trip to Haiti where we performed bread-and-butter surgeries like hernias, breast surgeries, and thyroidectomies. What impressed me most was the profound and immediate impact I saw on each surgical patient's life as opposed to medical patients who may have disease their entire lives. With surgery, a patient with an inguinal hernia that is large and debilitating can have surgery, and within a month be healed and again become the primary breadwinner for their family.

My life was changed. After this, the only question was what specialty of surgery would I choose? I did not have guidance and no one in my family worked in healthcare. I rotated through family medicine in rural Nebraska and had the privilege of working with a general surgeon who performed many different general surgeries including ruptured abdominal aortic aneurysms.

This is a weakening of the wall of the major blood vessel that supplies organs in the abdomen and lower body that advances to the point where the blood vessel bursts causing blood to leak into the abdomen.

This experience is why I pursued general surgery but at this time, I was not aware vascular surgery was an option. To be honest, I wanted to complete my residency in a warm climate because I did not want to shovel snow early in the mornings as we did in Nebraska. I was accepted at the Loma Linda University Medical Center in Southern California for residency. This was the perfect place for me.

My residency was great. It felt like we were all a family and that I belonged to a community. This was perfect since I did not have family in California. When I began my residency training, I disliked vascular surgery because vascular patients are so ill and sometimes their conditions were severe enough for them to be in danger of losing a leg or losing their lives.

As a junior resident, vascular surgery is difficult to understand because the patients have complicated and complex problems. For instance, learning to read angiograms, pictures of blood vessels flowing to and nourishing areas of the body, to determine reasons a patient has abnormal blood flow to body areas is difficult at first. With time and experience, understanding vascular diseases and diagnostic and treatment modalities becomes easier. At Loma Linda, we rotated through vascular surgery each year during the first four years of residency.

When I was a second-year resident rotating in vascular surgery, I did not consider vascular surgery as a career until I replaced a senior resident who was unable to complete his commitment to vascular surgery for one month. This was my second rotation in vascular that year.

Initially, I thought I was being punished. Why would they put me on vascular surgery again? I was a second-year resident in the role of a senior resident. It turned out to be the best experience I ever had.

One night, a patient came into the hospital with a

ruptured abdominal aortic aneurysm. I was on call with Dr. Sheela Patel. I called her and advised her of the patient's status and need for surgery. She replied, "Ok. Book it. Let's go." This meant for me to prepare the patient for surgery and make the necessary arrangements with the operating room.

I asked if she needed me to call a more senior resident or fellow and she asked, "Are you not going to be there?" I was shocked to learn she was comfortable doing the case with me. We performed the surgery together. I was in awe because typically this is a complicated case and the most senior resident is the person who assists the attending in this operation.

The next time I was on call, a patient presented with a type A dissection with associated limb ischemia. A bypass was indicated. A type A dissection occurs when a tear develops in the first part of the aorta, the largest vessel in the body, as it branches from the heart. In this case, occlusion (blockage) of the artery supplying blood to the arm occurred and needed repair.

The attending asked me to prep and drape and start dissecting the femoral artery and vein. I dissected and encircled the vessels the same way I saw my seniors do this and when I was finished, I asked if I should go to the other side. She looked up and said, "Wow, you are done? Yes, go to the other side." We worked well together, and I felt at home with the vascular team. They left a positive mark on me and I received so much support from them. One of the best technical surgeons I have ever worked with was our chief of vascular. Another surgeon, who was one of the most compassionate surgeons I knew and wanted to model my practice after, was there as well.

After these experiences, I wanted to train at the University of Oregon, Eugene, because this is where the chief trained, and he was amazing. I felt blessed when I matched in Oregon. My fellowship training was an amazing experience and again, I felt like I was part of the family. We did all we could for the patients as we worked well as a team.

One attending once said, "We may not agree on how to treat each individual case when we discuss them, but we do believe that whatever treatment we decide on is the best treatment for that patient. We don't cut corners or cut time, and no one is saying the patient is not a surgical candidate because we always do what is best for the patient." Of course, there were times patients would not benefit from surgery, but we made sure we exhausted all non-surgical options and provided the care that was in their best interest. I appreciated how the partners worked well and treated each other with respect where I trained.

I feel as a black female, there will always be challenges. There were no other black females in my program, but there were other females, and we had similar experiences. I remember being told to change my voice to make it softer and more pleasant. It seemed some felt my voice was harsh and I felt I was being criticized because I am female. I have always been concise and definitive, and this was not appreciated; the situation improved with time.

I remember one patient the urology service asked us to consult on. When I evaluated the patient, I determined they were ill enough to require intensive care unit (ICU) treatment. I transferred the patient to the surgical ICU and felt I acted in the patient's best interest by doing so.

Since I was unable to contact the chief resident, I spoke with another member of the urology team. When he discovered the patient was transferred to the SICU, he treated me meanly and told his attending what happened.

His attending discussed the situation with my attending, the chief of trauma. My attending reviewed the situation and realized I provided the proper care and made the right decision. He was objective and defended me. I was amazed when I heard this because this was an elderly white male physician who defended my actions. This does not happen very often. Having people advocating for you helps your career.

Confidence is an ongoing challenge for me, but I am becoming more confident as times passes. I never had the desire to be in academic surgery until my second year of fellowship training. Representation matters. We, as black females, do not have much representation. It is difficult to see where I am and where I wish to be because many times as black females, we must pave the way for ourselves and those coming after us. For instance, I never learned to write grants, but I am doing it. It is difficult, but I hear others agreeing it is difficult for them as well. I sometimes experience impostor syndrome and I combat these feelings by working hard, asking for help when I need it, and being humble. I tell myself, "Don't be afraid or feel ashamed to be yourself and you deserve to be there just as much as anybody else and maybe more."

As for my job, I spend half my time at the Veteran's Administration (VA) and the other half at the University Hospital because I am undecided about working full time for the VA or full time for the University Hospital.

I want to help VA patients because they are a vulnerable population. Veterans come to the VA for their care and I find it incredible to be able to serve those who served our country.

A typical week for me consists of two days seeing clinic patients and three days operating. This is split evenly between the VA and the University Hospital. We have residents and fellows in both programs. I enjoy teaching and mentoring students and surgical trainees.

My proudest moment is when I consider how we are trailblazing for ourselves and those to come. Everything we do is a huge accomplishment and forges a path for others. My parents have advanced degrees, but neither felt their degrees were as important as my medical degree. I have a twin brother and when I graduated from medical school, he graduated with his master's degree the same day. I attended his graduation in Lincoln, Nebraska, early in the morning so I could see him walk across the stage, and he came to Omaha to watch me walk across the stage. I do not think my parents have ever been prouder!

In the middle of all my chaos, I am still searching for balance. Some weeks are better than others. You must be intentional about it. For my future downtime, I have five books that have been on my list to read for a few years. I am trying to make time for them when I can enjoy reading non-medical books once again.

There are several people I would like to have dinner and talk with and hear their stories. First would be a dinner party with my mother, father, and grandparents so I can listen to their stories. I wish my grandparents could see me now. I feel I am my ancestors' dreams fulfilled. I would love to sit with Vivien Thomas because I imagine he felt the way we feel, the feelings of not belonging and inadequacy. I would love to hear how he felt throughout the process and how he would feel knowing that his name is now included in the name of the shunt he helped create (The Blalock-Thomas-Taussig Shunt) for 'blue babies,' babies born with four heart defects. Also, I would like to talk to myself when I was 20 years old. I do not regret anything, and I do not regret my course. Maybe I could have convinced myself to complete a master's degree in public health. It would be interesting to hear who I thought I was at that time. And, I would love to talk to my 70-year-old me!

My final words to all are, "You have got to see it before you BE it!"

"If the front side of the coin of success is the ability to set clear goals for yourself, then the flip side of the same coin is the ability to get yourself organized and work on your most valuable tasks, every minute of every day in order to achieve your goals. Your choices and decisions have combined to create your entire life to this moment. To change or improve your life in any way, you have to make new choices and new decisions that are more in alignment with who you really are and what you really want."
– Brian Tracy

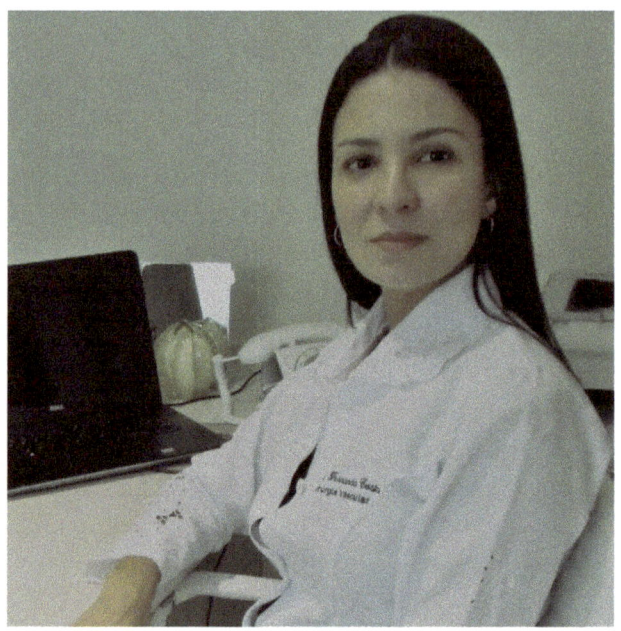

Dr. Fernanda Costa Sampaio Silva

Dr. Fernanda Costa Sampaio Silva is a vascular surgeon at the Centro Medico Hospital da Bahia, Department of Angiology and Vascular Surgery in Brazil, South America. She earned her medical degree from the Federal University of Bahia in Brazil and completed both general surgery and vascular surgery residencies at the Federal University of Bahia in Brazil and Ana Nery Hospital in Brazil. She is a member of the board of directors of the Brazilian Society of Angiology and Vascular Surgery (SBACV), regional Bahia and a member of the International Relations Committee, Society for Vascular Surgery (SVS).

Dr. Sampaio Silva is the daughter of a black father and a white mother. Unfortunately, in Brazil, there are still many remnants of the time of slavery. Racism is one of them. But she believes the greatest difficulty in being an Afro-descendant and wanting a medical career was economic limitation. In her country, she feels elementary and secondary education in public schools does not provide quality education. This makes it challenging for students applying to medical school. In the '80s and '90s, there was no quota policy at universities, so her parents had to work hard to pay for private education, otherwise, she would not have been able to fulfill her dreams of becoming a doctor.

Medicine is a prestigious profession in Brazil and difficult to achieve, which is why becoming a doctor was a great challenge. In Dr. Sampaio Silva's opinion, having professional freedom means not being afraid to deal with difficult situations. For this reason, she chose surgery, more specifically vascular surgery. She realized if she had the anatomical and technical knowledge about blood vessels, she would not be afraid to perform surgery on a human being.

Dr. Sampaio Silva has strong faith which maintains her confidence. She thinks becoming a doctor could only have been God's plan because looking at things in the natural realm, she would never have succeeded. When she investigated the paths her neighbors and childhood friends took, she realized they had different destinies than she. So, she is fully convinced that strength does not reside in her being, it comes from above.

At times along the way, Dr. Sampaio Silva struggled with impostor syndrome. It haunts her. Sometimes she feels she is in positions previously reached by rich, white people and grapples with thoughts that she does not belong where she is. Then, she takes a breath and remembers the reasons she is here. She asks herself, "Am I in leadership of any department?" And she answers, "Yes! And why did they choose me? Because I met all the requirements! Therefore, I am not an impostor!"

Dr. Sampaio Silva's greatest achievement so far was being selected as a committee member of a respected American society. No doctor in her specialty in her country has ever been selected for this position. And the best advice she ever received was, "No job, even if it is your dream, is worth your sanity." She had colleagues who committed suicide because they could not withstand the pressure of their own expectations.

To find balance, Dr. Sampaio Silva loves her husband and her son. Because she chose to have a husband and child, she makes sure she does not allow her career to absorb her. She constantly reviews her priorities, so she does not neglect them. And in her spare time, she is reading the article, *Leadership in American Surgery: Women are Rising to the Top*, recently published in the *Annals of Surgery* magazine.

Her father is the first of three people she would love to have dinner with and learn from. He died 10 years ago without seeing the results of his commitment to her career. He taught her to never give up. She would just like to say, "Thank you." Second is Rita Lobato Lopes, the first Brazilian female doctor. Dr. Sampaio Silva would like to hear what advice she would give her. And last would be Michael DeBakey, the pioneer in surgical procedures for treatment of defects and diseases of the cardiovascular system.

Words of wisdom Dr. Sampaio Silva would like to share with every reader are, "Do not let them judge you by appearance. Many may not call you doctor because you are black or have curly hair. But do not be ashamed to correct someone who confuses you with other professionals, such as a nurse or an assistant. Sometimes you will consider giving up. It is at this point you must rescue your roots and remember where you came from and how far you have come. Then keep walking. Have a life project beyond your career. Okay, you have become a surgeon and you have done a memorable job in society, but so what? Who are you outside the hospital? Do not lose your identity as a mother, wife, daughter, friend, and woman. It is to these places you will return when you feel overwhelmed and need to recharge your batteries to continue your career!"

CHAPTER SEVENTEEN
Ophthalmology Surgery

Ophthalmologists are physicians specializing in the comprehensive medical and surgical care of the eyes and vision. Ophthalmologists are the only practitioners medically trained to diagnose and treat all eye and visual problems including vision services (glasses and contacts) and provide treatment and prevention of medical disorders of the eye including surgery.

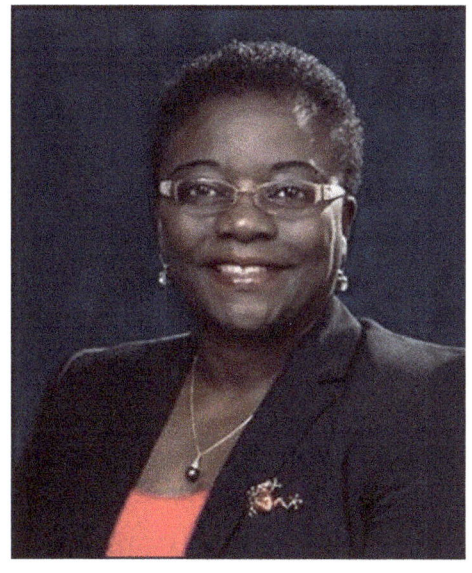

Dr. Sade Kosoko-Lasaki

Dr. Sade Kosoko-Lasaki is associate vice provost of the Health Sciences Multicultural and Community Affairs (HS-MACA) Department at Creighton University in Omaha, Nebraska. She is also a tenured professor of ophthalmology surgery and preventive medicine and public health at the Creighton University School of Medicine. She is co-founder and co-director of the Center for Promoting Health & Health

Equality.

Dr. Kosoko-Lasaki is a dynamite lady and has accomplished much in her 40-plus-year career. She is passionate about her work and, despite numerous obstacles along the way, she persisted and made a name for herself in her discipline. She completed her medical school in Nigeria and trained in ophthalmology at the University of Glasgow in Glasgow, Scotland.

She migrated to the United States and completed another residency at Howard University in Washington, D.C., and a subspecialty fellowship in glaucoma at Johns Hopkins University in Baltimore, Maryland.

She is a wife and mother of three, a stepmother of three, and a grandmother of three. She has been awarded multi-million-dollar grants for her research initiatives. She authored two major textbooks for ophthalmology and has authored multiple book chapters as well as numerous papers for publication. Her CV (resume) is 24 pages long. She is the epitome of an academic surgeon powerhouse.

Dr. Kosoko-Lasaki is passionate about eliminating health care disparities as well as minority health development and has won multiple national and international awards for her research in glaucoma, a disease of the eye resulting from increased pressure in the eye. Part of her research focuses on increasing minorities in the healthcare workforce. At Creighton University, she oversees the recruitment of disadvantaged students to the health sciences and mentors these students to retain them.

She lectures around the country and the world on cultural proficiency and health disparity issues. She focuses on the promotion of pipeline programs that prepare and support disadvantaged students from grade four through health professional schools so they may become successful health care providers.

She served as a consultant for the United Nations Children's Education Fund (UNICEF), the United States Agency for International Development (USAID), and Helen Keller

International in West African countries, the Caribbean, and Asia. She expanded her outreach efforts to the Dominican Republic screening for glaucoma, performing eye surgeries, and combating childhood vitamin A deficiency.

Dr. Kosoko-Lasaki was instrumental in creating Glaucoma Initiative in the U.S. Virgin Islands, Nigeria, Rural Nebraska, Iowa, and Kansas screening of more than 20,000 individuals for glaucoma.

This is Dr. Kosoko-Lasaki's story in her words.

I was born in Sapele, Nigeria. My father, Dr. Babalola, was an optometrist, one of the first in Nigeria. He attended university in the United Kingdom and afterward returned to Nigeria where he opened his optometry practice. Before going to the United Kingdom, he was a pharmacist. Thus, I was exposed to medicine early in childhood.

When we were young, my sister and I went to our father's clinic and helped his patients select frames for glasses. I grew up loving optometry and told my father I wanted to be an optometrist like him. He told me if I wanted to practice with him someday it would be best if I was an ophthalmologist because I would be able to perform surgical procedures of the eye, which he was not able to do as an optometrist.

I was 13 years old and never knew there was such a field of medicine. I discovered that to become an ophthalmologist, I needed to attend medical school. I also realized I needed to work hard in school to earn excellent grades because this is a requirement for acceptance into medical school. At age 16, I was accepted into one of the premier medical schools at the University of Ibadan in Nigeria, Africa. I graduated from medical school at 22 years old.

After completing my national service at one of the largest hospitals for ophthalmology in Nigeria, an opportunity presented to apply for a scholarship to train in Scotland to specialize in ophthalmology. In some countries, doctors are required to complete one- or two-years work as a general practitioner in government hospitals after completing medical school. In 1979,

I attended the University of Glasgow, Glasgow, Scotland, and completed my training in 1982. I planned to return to Nigeria to practice with my father.

I met my first husband when I was studying abroad in Scotland. He was from the United States. This is how my path took me to the United States after finishing my training in Scotland.

It was difficult for anyone from outside the United States to be accepted for a position to train in ophthalmology at that time. I started from the beginning in terms of residency training. It took me seven years to achieve my goal of becoming an ophthalmologist. While waiting for acceptance, I strengthened my application by earning a master's degree in public health. I worked as a consultant for the WHO, UNICEF through the Helen Keller Foundation. Through my research, we were awarded a USAID grant in St. Lucia in the Caribbean for research on glaucoma.

With a stronger application, I was accepted into Howard University, Washington D.C., for my residency in ophthalmology. After finishing residency, I was accepted to Johns Hopkins University, Baltimore, Maryland, for a fellowship in glaucoma.

I had two children before starting residency. My first child was born in 1983 and my second child was born in 1984. My youngest child was born in 1987. My children have always been my priority; even when I traveled internationally for research, I was able to take my children with me. I always made certain to ask for childcare as part of the package. Sometimes, I took my children to my parents in Nigeria for care because I became a single mother shortly after my third child was born. I have never used my children as an excuse for not getting my work done. I completed my work two to three days before due dates because I could never predict what could happen with the children. If they became ill, I was concerned this may cause me not to be able to complete my assignments or presentations.

I hired a live-in nanny to help during the week while I was in residency. I generally woke at 6 a.m. to prepare for the day. My day started with spending time with God. I took the train to work so I could read and complete my assignments. I worked moonlighting so I could afford to pay for a live-in nanny. This meant I had no days off because whenever I was not in residency training, I worked my moon-lighting shifts. My children were in bed by 8:30 p.m. every night so I was able to read and complete my assignments, which I usually worked on until 1 a.m.

When I finished my fellowship, I returned to Howard University in Washington, D.C., where I worked on faculty for 10 years before moving to Omaha, Nebraska, where I have been for 20 years.

Academic surgery does not pay as well as private practice, so one must have a love and passion for it to choose this career path.

I recommend young women have specific goals to accomplish their career. For me, I knew I wanted to advance from assistant professor of surgery to associate professor of surgery within five years. The only way I would be able do this was by having scientific papers published in peer-review journals. I was disciplined. My day went from 8 a.m. to 5 p.m. each day, even on days I finished seeing clinic patients by 2 p.m. I used the extra time to do research, work on projects, and write papers. When you are ready to advance from associate professor to full professor, you need to add community service and committee memberships to your curriculum vitae.

A word of caution, you need to learn to say, "No," to committees and responsibilities that do not serve you well for advancement. It is easy to say, "Yes," to every committee you are asked to be a part of because you are happy you are being asked. But it is easy to become overwhelmed by too many responsibilities. I made a point to choose only three committees to be a member of at any given time.

Unlike many who pass-up opportunities because a job may not be in an ideal location or they do not want to be someplace where there is snow, I will go anywhere a great opportunity presents. I have never seen myself as a professional woman, but I am a professional. I learned early on that I am my own best advocate. I am my own champion and have learned to surround myself with people who champion me. For instance, my second husband has been a supportive partner who believes in me and wants me to be my best self.

My advice is to always be yourself because it does not matter what titles you have. At the end of the day, you are a physician and your calling is to serve patients. Your patients trust you to take care of them the best way you know how.

As I scrub my hands before each surgery, I pray for God's guidance. We are human and at times we become prideful of our abilities. I always ask God to help me remain humble and I know that God is in control in all situations. I have experienced complications, but the Lord always gives me the serenity to identify my complications and the humility to admit to them.

Part of my humility is that I know when to call for help or when to refer my patients to someone I feel will provide better care. I always tell my patients that if they have reservations about me as their surgeon, they should tell me, and I will find someone else to care for them. My mentor at Johns Hopkins taught me that I must remember every patient I operate on because they trusted me and took a chance on me. Another thing he said was to always, always be available to my patients such that when they call me, I take time to speak with them because they trust me.

When it came to finding balance, I took long walks with my children when they were young. I walked while they rode their bicycles. I do water aerobics two to three times a week and enjoy long walks to this day. I am extremely disciplined about what I eat. After turning 40, my metabolism slowed, so anything I put in my mouth I ask myself, "Is this food helping me or killing me?"

I visit my physician annually for health check-ups and make certain my cancer screening tests, my pap smear, mammogram, and colonoscopy, are up to date. I do not treat myself; I have my doctor who treats me. I make a point to keep my mind and emotions healthy and do not allow people or things around me that do not make me happy.

Currently, I am reading a book about military men who played a big role in the independence of Nigeria.

I have a mentoring group for undergraduate students on Facebook. I research articles and post them on Facebook for my group, so I read a great deal.

I also have another mentoring group for practicing physicians to help them avoid burnout, which has the added benefit of keeping me up to date with literature about burnout and physician wellness. Between these two groups, I read a great deal. I am busy, but I love the life I have.

"I alone cannot change the world, but I can cast a stone across the water to create many ripples." – Mother Teresa

CHAPTER EIGHTEEN
ENT Surgery

An otolaryngologist-head and neck surgeon is a physician who has been prepared by an accredited residency program to provide comprehensive medical and surgical care of patients with diseases and disorders that affect the ears, the respiratory and upper alimentary systems, and related structures of the head and neck.

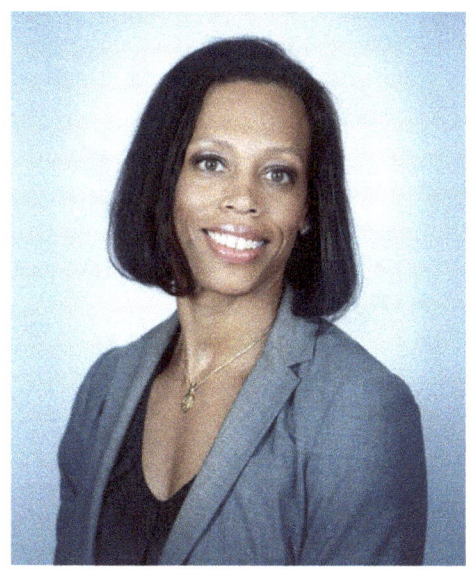

Dr. Gina Jefferson

Dr. Gina Jefferson is an associate professor and chief of the division of head and neck oncologic and microvascular surgery, as well as vice-chair of education, in the Department of Otolaryngology and Communicative Sciences at the University of Mississippi Medical Center, Jackson, Mississippi.

She earned her medical degree from Case Western Reserve University School of Medicine, Cleveland, Ohio, and completed her residency in otolaryngology head and neck surgery at Loma Linda University Medical Center, Loma Linda, California.

She continued to the department of otolaryngology, University of Miami, Miami, Florida, to complete her fellowship training in head and neck surgical oncology and microvascular reconstruction.

Dr. Jefferson is certified by the American Board of Otolaryngology. She specializes in head and neck surgical oncology, microvascular reconstruction, and trans-oral robotic surgery. This includes the surgical management of adult oropharyngeal and supraglottic tumors and obstructive sleep apnea.

Her interests focus on research of head and neck cancers including patient outcomes, quality of life, and health care disparities among head and neck cancer patients. Dr. Jefferson has several articles in peer-reviewed publications and has presented at numerous national meetings including the American College of Surgeons, the American Academy of Otolaryngology, and the National Medical Association.

Dr. Jefferson grew up in Cleveland, Ohio. She and her sister were the first in their immediate family to attend college. Her sister has a Ph.D. Their parents encouraged them to be well-educated so Dr. Jefferson and her sister would enjoy a better life than they had. Dr. Jefferson had no aspirations of becoming a physician when she was a child but was proficient in math and science, and she participated in track. Because of her ability in track, she was granted a scholarship to Purdue University in Fort Wayne, Indiana, to study engineering. When she interacted with other athletes, she closely watched how they recovered after being injured. Their recovery was tremendous, and they were able to perform again despite their injuries. This fascinated her and she considered a career as a biomedical engineer.

As Dr. Jefferson worked toward her master's degree in biomedical engineering, she realized she is a people person and wanted to do something that allowed her to work with others on a team. Her first project was building a device that allowed children with cerebral palsy to swim. As she interacted with each child, she realized she really enjoyed working with children. This was when she decided she wanted to become a doctor. Initially, she thought her road would lead her to medical school to become an orthopedic surgeon.

During her third year in medical school, she considered gynecologic oncology but quickly changed her mind. Dr. Jefferson's mother was diagnosed with breast cancer when she was 37 years old. This made her consider breast surgical oncology, but she was not passionate about general surgery.

After medical school, she matched at Howard University in Washington, D.C., for her general surgery residency. It was during her residency that she was exposed to the ENT (ear/nose/and throat) specialty. As a first and second-year resident, she rotated on the endocrine surgery service. Dr. Jefferson enjoyed this her first year, but it was not until her second year of residency that she fell in love with ENT. She chose to complete a year doing research after the second year of general surgery residency and then matched with the Charles Drew Medical Center, Los Angeles, California for her residency in ENT.

During her second year of residency in ENT, her hospital (Charles Drew Medical Center) closed. Dr. Jefferson was forced to find another program. She was accepted at Loma Linda University Medical Center, Loma Linda, California, to finish her training.

Being the only female did not faze her; she was grateful for a program to train her. She was made chief resident in her chief year and her training was exceptional. Dr. Jefferson's residency at Howard prepared her for success in her current training and career because she worked with surgeons who looked like her and who were brilliant! They were great teachers and the residents, in turn, worked extremely hard and made sure they were prepared for rounds and operations.

Dr. Jefferson aspires to become a department chair

because she wants to be able to give back and help others who look like her and are coming up the ranks. She wants young women thinking of a career in medicine to know mentoring and sponsorship are important for professional growth. And she thinks confidence comes in your own institution where you develop relationships with other doctors and specialties. It is important to be engaged in your own system. When you deliver presentations at meetings, the key is to be well-prepared. Always be well-prepared for cases, for rounds, for the clinic, for whatever it is you are doing. Preparation is key!

Dr. Jefferson is convinced that finding a mentor is important. Find someone who is doing what you want to do. For those interested in pursuing a fellowship, she wants them to know they do not have to consider the specialty for which they are specifically trained. Fellowship training opens more doors and the ability to carve-out a personal niche, even in general practice. Fellowship allows the choice to do private practice or academic surgery.

Also, Dr. Jefferson advises her mentees to seek opportunities, shadow doctors, make early connections to familiarize yourself with medicine, always work hard because you never know what it is you will end up wanting to do, and do not be afraid to ask questions.

Dr. Jefferson credits her success to God. Her faith is important to her. For her, her time spent with God has evolved in a more structured way. Now that she has more control of her time, she makes a point to spend time with God in the morning before starting her day. She is grateful for her life and for the fact she is blessed to do what she loves to do. Dr. Jefferson works at a job she loves so much; not many people can say this. In residency, she had her Bible app on her phone and whenever she had time to read, she read and prayed, even in the car on her way to work or home. Finding time may be difficult, but it is important to try.

Now, in a typical work week, she spends three to four days in the operating room and one day, sometimes one-and-a-half days, seeing clinic patients. She spends half a day or one day doing administrative work.

If Dr. Jefferson could do one surgery, and only one surgery, every day for the rest of her life it would be microvascular free tissue transfers because it gives her the ability to reconstruct in many different ways. This procedure is when a block of skin, tissue, muscle, or bone is removed from a donor site and attached to the area in need of reconstruction. Dr. Jefferson must use a microscope to see and connect the tiny blood vessels in the free flap to the blood vessels at the recipient site. Very thin sutures (stitches) are used to join these tiny blood vessels.

In the operating room, Dr. Jefferson often plays "Black Eyed Peas" radio.

Three people Dr. Jefferson would want to have dinner with and learn from are Nelson Mandela, because of his perseverance and service to others; Oprah Winfrey, who wonderfully took advantage of the American dream and overcame some overwhelming odds and is the epitome of doing what you love and giving back to others; and Misty Copeland, because everyone told her she could not be a ballerina because she started so late. Not only is she a ballerina, but she is the best ballerina. She is the first African American woman promoted to principal dancer in the prestigious American Ballet Theater's 75-year history. She is pretty amazing.

Dr. Jefferson's final words of encouragement are, "You can do anything you set your mind to. Enjoy the process and do not forget to give back!"

"If you can't fly, then run. If you can't run, then walk. If you can't walk, then crawl, but whatever you do, you have to keep moving forward."
–Martin Luther King, Jr.

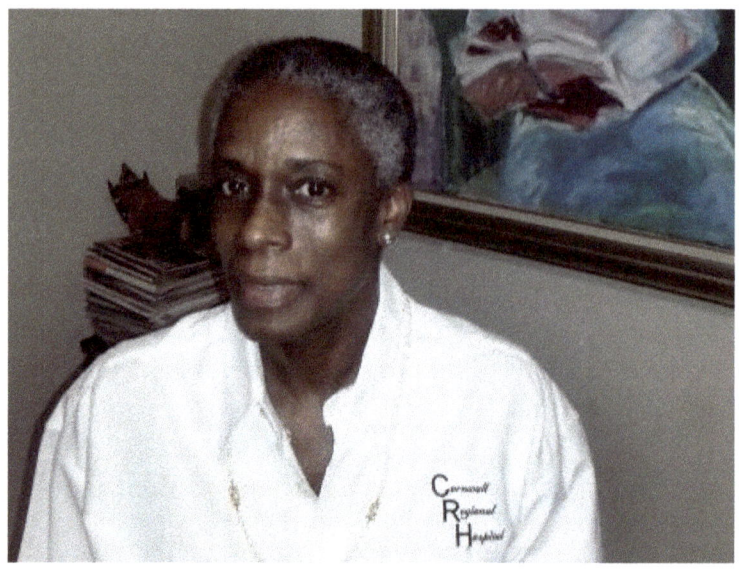

Dr. Barbara Grandison

Dr. Barbara Grandison grew up in a family with many siblings in Spanish Town, Jamaica. She attended primary school in Spanish Town and then commuted every day to high school in Kingston, Jamaica. While in high school, she was in girl guides and rangers (girl scouts), and there was a program where the girls could be candy stripers at the hospital to help sick people. They also visited a home for mentally disabled children. There, they interacted with children with various congenital and mental disorders. It was at this time Dr. Grandison became interested in their care and decided she wanted to be a psychiatrist. When she discovered she needed to go to medical school to become a psychiatrist, she applied to the university with her friends because this made it fun and not stressful. Dr. Grandison was accepted to complete the preliminary courses at the university in preparation for medical school. She did well her first year and was accepted to medical school.

Dr. Grandison was not the best student in the class, but she worked hard and graduated from medical school. During medical school in her country, they were able do locums where they worked and were paid. Dr. Grandison did locums in the ENT (ear/nose/throat) department. This was when she realized she enjoyed this work and chose ENT as a specialty.

When Dr. Grandison graduated from medical school, she spent part of her internship training in ENT and the other time training in chest medicine. She began her ENT residency after her internship.

She was fortunate to have a great mentor during her residency at the University of West Indies, Jamaica, who helped her grow as a physician and surgeon. Dr. Grandison chose to work in public service, at a government hospital, in Montego Bay, Jamaica, where there were no ENT specialists and amazingly created a new ENT program. It was extremely challenging to start a program, so in the beginning she did everything on her own because there were no interns or residents. Dr. Grandison had a supportive anesthesiologist that made those first few years as the only ENT specialist more manageable.

It was great to watch the program grow. Now they have three consultant ENT surgeons and the program trains residents. Dr. Grandison also has a private practice she opened in 1987 at the same time she began working in public service. This is going well. If she could do one surgery for the rest of her career it would be tonsillectomies and thyroidectomies. Wait, this is two operations!

The challenges Dr. Grandison faced in the Caribbean were not due to being a female because women have been doing many male-dominated jobs for a long time. There are instances she passed on opportunities that could have advanced her career, but she chose to prioritize her family. Challenges were more institutional based, such as shortage of resources, manpower, and supplies, not discrimination or sexism.

To build confidence, Dr. Grandison advises new doctors to read about patients' conditions and treatments and about the operations and discuss everything with mentors. She felt empowered because her mentors empowered her and guided her.

Dr. Grandison tells her residents there is no substitute for being well-prepared. Know everything about the patient. It is not about experiencing complications because complications will happen. It is about how you prepare for surgery, how you prepare your patients for surgery, and how you recognize complications and deal with them before they escalate.

She does not want her learning doctors to be afraid because something adverse may happen, but Dr. Grandison wants them to think about how to fix problems when they present. She welcomes suggestions. So, if she does something one way and someone shares how they find another way that works, she is willing to add to her armamentarium.

Dr. Grandison also coaches learning doctors to be willing to do what is required, sometimes more than what their job description is. Do whatever it takes to make things flow smoothly. The priority is the patients. It is important to be compassionate. Take time to talk and listen to patients. Dr. Grandison always treats her patients as she would her loved ones. She has a 33-year-old son.

Final words shared by Dr. Grandison are, "It is been a journey of learning and a journey of independence and dependence. Pave a way for others and after you finish your tour of duty you may end up being the patient. So it is important that what you leave behind will serve everyone so that even the least among us can receive great care."

"I am grateful to those who did not take a chance on me. They, especially, sparked the fire that ignited my resilience. It is because of them that I learned how to adjust my sails and stay in the race. Each of us men and women will encounter challenges great and small in our careers. General Patton once said that he did not measure a man's success by how high he climbs but how high he bounces when he hits the bottom. Let's help future generations of surgeons male and female bounce higher."
– Julie Freischlag, MD

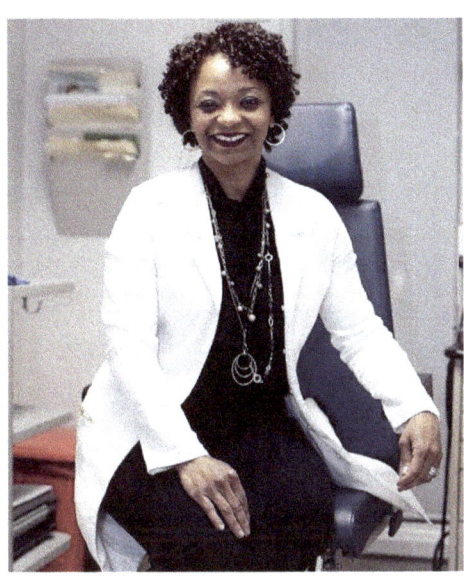

Dr. Tonia Farmer

Dr. Tonia Farmer completed her medical school training at the Virginia Commonwealth University Medical College of Virginia in Richmond, Virginia, where she was inducted into the honor society, Alpha Omega Alpha. She remained there for her residency in Otolaryngology (ENT) and was the first female ever accepted into its residency program.

Otolaryngologist/Head and Neck Surgeon Dr. Farmer practices in Warren, Ohio. She owns the world-renowned Lippy Group for ear, nose, and throat care and the Lippy Surgery Center. In addition to her practice, she launched a company in 2018 called Salt Me! Her company specializes in Himalayan sea salt sinus and body care products, as well as provides easy to understand health and wellness education.

This is Dr. Farmer's story in her words.

The defining moment that made me choose medicine as a career was when my twin sister was diagnosed with osteosarcoma (bone cancer) when we were seven years old. My desire to become a doctor started with this experience and her being in and out of the hospital. How her doctors cared for her and our family impacted me greatly. I knew one day I wanted to be a doctor so I could do this for other people. Sonia died when we were nine years old. Though it has been a little more than 40 years since her passing, she has been the driving force behind my perseverance and success. I wanted to be a doctor for her, too.

One of the greatest challenges I faced during my journey was impostor syndrome. I did not know it had a name. I suffered from this when I was in residency and as a new attending. I battled feelings of not deserving my position because I was the first female and only black person in my residency program.

There were instances when I felt as if patients were looking past me because I was black. One example is when I was leading my team on rounds as a chief resident and a Caucasian patient refused to address me when speaking. This patient addressed their questions to the junior resident, a white male. The patient did this despite this junior resident redirecting him to me, the most experienced and senior member of the team. I experienced different feelings when I walked into a room with a Caucasian patient than I did entering a room with a black patient. I felt appreciated by people who looked like me.

There was an instance in training when a patient was blatantly racist. My attending removed me from this patient's care. He advocated for me so I would not be subjected to this type of treatment.

Another challenge I faced was my image was not accepted. I planned a vacation to a Caribbean island and had my hair specially braided. It is helpful for black women to keep our hair braided when we plan to be in water for long periods of time. When I returned from vacation, an attending told me my hair style was not professional because it was braided, even though my braids were professionally styled and neat.

The expectation was my hair be styled straight. This showed me I could not be myself and was forced to conform to society's idea of what is professional when it comes to black women's hair.

For the remainder of my training and into my early years

as an attending, I wore my hair straight. Now, however, I wear my hair natural and am comfortable this way. It may seem like an insignificant topic, but for black women, these are some of the challenges we face.

Sometimes black women must conform and wear their hair straight or in weaves and wigs to be accepted into positions. Some have the courage to wear their hair natural once they are established in their jobs and can make their own decisions without it impacting their career trajectory.

In ENT, I felt my greatest challenge was being black rather than being female. This field has many females, but a small number of blacks. I had excellent training and I did not feel I was treated differently from my male colleagues in terms of training opportunities. I feel ENT is a gentler surgical field to women compared to other surgical specialties.

A typical workday begins with making sure my children are ready for school in the morning before I go to the office. I need to be at work earlier on days I perform surgery. Those days my husband takes over the task of getting our children ready to go. We have our specific roles with the children. I take care of the clothes and hair for the girls and my husband makes them a hot breakfast every morning. I am usually home by 6 or 7 p.m. on days I have surgery and earlier when I see clinic patients.

I would say the secret sauce to my success in life is surrounding myself with mentors and a strong support system. While going through my schooling and training I learned I needed cheerleaders to help me along who were also experiencing what I was or who had experienced it already.

I have a woman named Betty Golden, who, along with her husband, were pivotal in mentoring my husband and me in our marriage. For us, it was important to have a Christian couple as mentors for a godly marriage. They have been such a blessing to us.

I am a member of Jack and Jill of America, Inc. This organization for mothers with children ages 2-19 is dedicated to nurturing future African American leaders by strengthening children through leadership development, volunteer services, philanthropic giving, and civic duty.

This organization provides a great support system and I have another mother who understands the struggles of parenting. Her support has helped greatly.

My family keeps me grounded. Growing up, my main pillars of support where my mother, grandmother, and aunt, and when I married, my husband became another major support person.

As I have grown older, my support system has grown. I honestly believe in the African proverb that "It takes a village to raise a child." I am convinced it takes a village for a woman to become the best version of herself. Even though my twin sister is not with us, she is forever in my heart.

Finding balance is always a challenge. I work awfully hard because being in a private practice means I am a business owner. The work is never done. Gradually, I have learned to manage my time more efficiently and not feel guilty for not being able to do everything. I wear many hats in life. I am a wife, a mother of three girls, a daughter, and a doctor. I constantly check how I am doing in all these areas of my life. There is no way I will always have everything balanced.

In addition to my private practice, I started a company. Let me begin by saying that I love Himalayan sea salt! As you know, I am a board-certified otolaryngologist/head and neck surgeon (or ENT doctor) and I care for patients with sinus problems. Living in Ohio is good for my business because there are many patients with sinus problems here.

One of my patients introduced me to salt therapy (halotherapy) because she found it improved her chronic sinus symptoms. When I examined her sinuses with a scope, her sinus mucosa was healthy and appeared to be the healthiest I had ever seen it.

She shared how she began salt therapy sessions at Salt Sensations USA, LLC in Boardman, Ohio. I contacted the owner, Tracy Prizant, and visited her business. I experienced a salt therapy session with some of my staff members and was convinced that salt therapy was not only a growing spa treatment but also a beneficial, natural therapeutic option for my patients.

I spent hours securing and reviewing clinical research studies from Europe on the use of dry, aerosolized, inhaled Himalayan sea salt. These studies supported the benefit of salt therapy to improve respiratory and dermatological disorders.

I began recommending salt therapy to my patients as an adjunctive treatment to manage their upper and lower respiratory problems. I was interested to see how well salt therapy would work for my patients and how I could incorporate Himalayan sea salt into quality body and sinus care products that could be used at home. *Salt Me!* was born!

My love for entrepreneurship started early in life. During my surgical residency, I created a small business specializing in decorative, customized picture frames. It was a great DIY stress-reliever and allowed me to make a few extra dollars to help my tight budget. I have dabbled in other things along the way, including a party planning business I also do on the side. I really enjoy it, but I have not had much financial success from this because each job is usually a favor for my friends and family. But I must say, I do enjoy planning a great party and I am still considering making it an official business someday. In 2018, I launched Salt Me! This business has been doing well financially.

I enjoy success as an entrepreneur by co-owning the world-renowned Lippy Group for ENT and Lippy Surgery Center. The Lippy Surgery Center is a multi-specialty ambulatory surgery center established in 2008. We have delivered quality surgical and post-operative care to thousands of adults and children from around the world. Hearing-impaired clients have visited from all over the United States, Canada, and as far away as Israel for life-changing surgical procedures to improve and restore hearing.

Surgical specialties offered at The Lippy Surgery Center include procedures for eyes, ears, nose, and the throat as well as both functional and cosmetic plastic surgeries. Specialties related to ears include middle and inner-ear implants, bone anchored hearing aids, and cochlear implants. We regularly perform pediatric ear, nose, and throat procedures and maintain an outstanding safety record. We offer vocal and functional nasal surgeries as well as sinus procedures using high-tech CT guidance for optimal results.

Giving back by supporting small business owners is also important to me. They inspire me to keep growing. *Salt Me!* is a natural extension of my medical practice and allows me to put my desire to help others into action. It has become a family business because my three girls, Sonia, Simone, and Sanaa, as well as my husband Casey, provide the wind beneath my wings.

People I would like to have dinner with and learn from are first, Barack Obama. When I think of him, I think of grace under fire. Regardless of who he was dealing with, he was exemplary in the way he dealt with them. I want to know what made him walk with grace the eight years he was in office and dealt with racism and disrespect. I want to know how he managed to keep a level head and remain humble with all the accolades and praise. And, Harriet Tubman. When I think of her, I think of the phrase, "For such a time as this." She was born for the purpose of leading people out of slavery. Nothing deterred her from what she knew she had to do to bring freedom to others after she found freedom. She went back time and again. I would want to sit down and talk to her and glean small pieces of her strength and determination. Lastly, I would love to sit and have dinner with my twin sister, Sonia. When she was diagnosed with cancer, she knew she was going to die. My mother brought her home because the doctors told her there was nothing more they could do for her in the hospital. I remember that day. Sonia, who had her entire leg amputated and had multiple lung surgeries to remove cancer that spread there, was on home oxygen and could not breathe.

On the day she died, June 17, 1979, she said, "Mom call the ambulance because I can't breathe, and I am going to die tonight." She wrote a poem three months before she died. I have her poem on my wall, and I miniaturized it and laminated it and carry it in my wallet with me. She had the faith of a mustard seed. I want to sit and talk with her because at the time of her death, I did not understand her faith and what was going on. I want to know where her faith came from. How did it feel for her to know that she was leaving this earth and going to be with the Lord? I want her to see and know how much her life has meant to my life. I am who I am, and the doctor I am, for my patients because of her life. I want to be the kind of doctor who is loving and compassionate; the way her doctors were with her. Here is the poem:

> February 29, 1979
> <u>My prayer</u>
> The Lord is our savior
> We trust in Him. We love Him
> You should pray to Him
> He can see you and hear you
> Everyone in the whole wide world loves Him
> Some people do not love God and do not believe in Him
> But I know I do
> When you pray and ask God for something
> You may not get it; God will wait until He sees you are ready for what you want
> And sometimes you may not get it
> But do not worry, God may think that you do not need it
> Whoever does not believe in God
> I will try to pray for you, for anyone
>   Sonia

My final words of encouragement are, "Do NOT accept other people's opinions about yourself. Always command YOUR future to achieve success. I believe in the 5 P's: Positioning can be Painful but is always Purposeful to Prepare you for your Place. This means that at times you must go through difficulties, but you must persevere because each difficult experience is preparing you for your success.

"You've got to follow your passion. You've got to figure out what it is you love—who you really are. And have the courage to do that. I believe that the only courage anybody ever needs is the courage to follow your own dreams."
– Oprah Winfrey

CHAPTER NINETEEN
Plastics and Reconstructive Surgery

Plastics and reconstructive surgery deals with the repair, reconstruction, or replacement of physical defects of form or function involving the skin, musculoskeletal system, cranio and maxillofacial structures, hand, extremities, breast and trunk, and external genitalia. It uses aesthetic surgical principles not only to improve undesirable qualities of normal structures but also in all reconstructive procedures as well.

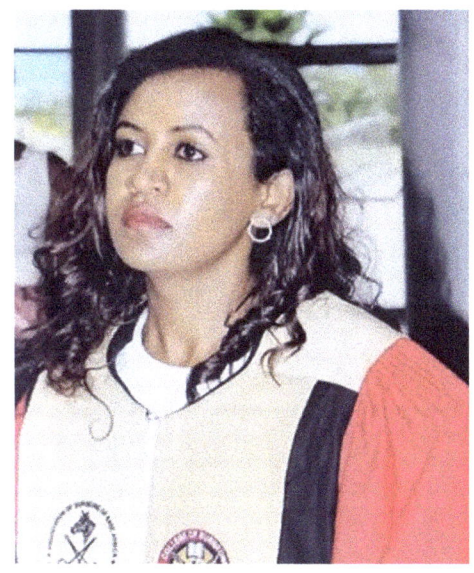

Dr. Metasebia Worku Abebe

Dr. Metasebia Worku Abebe earned her medical degree at Addis Ababa University in Ethiopia, Africa. She completed her two years of national service required in Ethiopia after completing medical school as a general medical practitioner at Saint Paul Millennium Medical College in Addis Ababa, Ethiopia. She also earned a Master of Public Health (MPH) at Addis Continental Institute of Public Health in Addis Ababa, during the time she completed her national service. She was accepted for her general surgery internship and a plastics and reconstructive surgery residency at Addis Ababa University. She is currently a consultant plastic and reconstructive surgeon at Saint Paul Millennium Medical College in Addis Ababa, Ethiopia.

This is Dr. Metasebia Worku Abebe's story in her own words.

Persistence and hard work were my strongest steppingstones as a surgeon. As the younger of two daughters of hard-working middle-class parents who prioritized education, I had a wonderful support system at home. I went to an all-girls school where I competed with other hard-working girls striving to succeed. This produced unwavering confidence in myself. I have always known I can achieve anything I want to achieve if I put the necessary effort and time into it.

My journey in medical school, as anyone who has experienced any extremely competitive and demanding environment knows, was far from smooth. There will be times when you think you have given all it takes, but the results are not satisfactory. This requires even more determination and effort.

As with many higher-education programs, I feel medical school is a male-dominated field and surgery is even more so. You come across many personalities in your schooling as well as your workplace that will attribute your achievements to your gender rather than your commitment or hard work. It is important to push through all these hurdles and not lose sight of the goals you set for yourself.

I was one of the five female general surgery residents accepted into a program that accepted 30 residents per year. I knew surgery was my passion, but I also knew it would be demanding and I had to be focused, so this is what I did.

As a female in an environment not accustomed to having women around, I felt I needed to do twice as much work to balance my work and personal life, but it is possible, and I made it. I feel you will have role models you look up to, colleagues that lift you and support you, and there will be nay-sayers who will try to discourage you. If you put your focus, determination, and hard work towards your goals, you can and will achieve them.

What I have told myself from an early age is, "You are doing well, but there is always room for improvement. You can do it. Push through!"

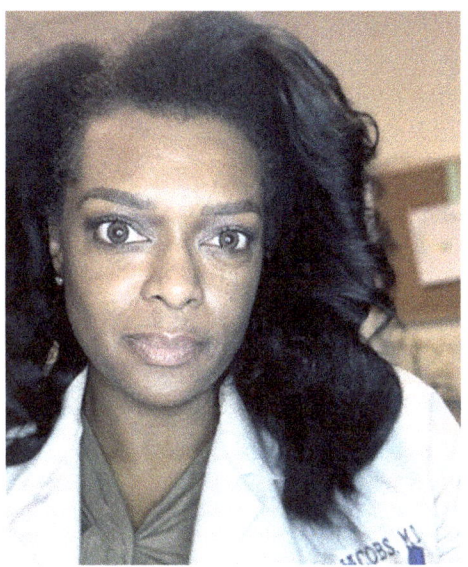

Dr. Sharone' M. Jacobs

Dr. Sharone' M. Jacobs graduated from Duke University, Durham, North Carolina, earning a bachelor of science in biology and a minor in chemistry. She received her medical degree at the Louisiana State University School of Medicine in New Orleans, Louisiana. She completed her internship and residency in general surgery at New York-Presbyterian Queens hospital in Flushing, New York. She is an associate fellow of the American College of Surgeons.

Dr. Jacobs's story is a testament to the fact that your career may not go exactly as you imagined at times, but in the end, it is the best thing that ever happened to you.

This is Dr. Jacobs' story in her words.

I grew up in New Iberia, Louisiana, with a population of

about 40,000 people. I had a good mixture of friends and experiences, which was much different than where I lived in New York for most of my adult life. I was enrolled in the honors program and did well in high school. I was a well-rounded student and involved in many extracurricular activities.

Initially, I aspired to become an attorney, so over one summer I had a job with a family friend who was an attorney in town. I worked at his office helping with faxing, filings, and occasionally researching cases at the courthouse. I loved it and thought I might enjoy practicing corporate law.

My first year in college, I studied biology with my boyfriend who was interested in medicine. Anatomy lab was love at first dissection! From there, I volunteered at hospitals over summer breaks in college. I was hooked from that point on and knew I wanted to be a physician.

Everything was easy initially. Undergraduate and medical school were a breeze, relatively speaking. Reality hit in surgical residency. This is when I encountered obstacles. To be honest, the first two years as a junior resident were heaven. I loved everything about surgery and my training. The challenges were when I became a senior resident, when the weight of my clinical decisions was more imperative.

It took a while to build confidence. I feel confidence is built with time and comes when you realize you are good enough. I took two years off from clinical work to conduct research in a plastic surgery laboratory at Columbia. I was challenged when I returned to my surgical residency, and it took time to regain my confidence because my skills were rusty. I suffered from impostor syndrome after finishing residency and was working locum jobs where I was the only available surgeon. To conquer impostor syndrome, you must get out of your own way and keep believing in yourself. I knew I was trained to handle almost anything. It is helpful to learn to block out the self-doubt.

Then, amazingly enough, an opportunity presented in wound care. I worked with Vohra Wound Physicians initially, then went on to work at Montefiore Hospital in New York. I worked in the vascular surgery department. I managed the hyperbaric clinic and did administrative work for about four years before I received a flyer recruiting hair restoration surgeons. I usually discarded such solicitation, however, this one caught my interest because secretly, I wanted to have eyebrow restoration myself.

I responded and the rest is history! I started my hair restoration career in our Manhattan, New York, office before moving to Philadelphia to manage this office. I love what I do! Not only do I wake up excited (most days) about transforming someone's life, but my schedule also affords me time to spend with my daughter. Currently I arrive at work at 7:30 a.m. and typically perform 2-3 cases a day. I finish about 5 p.m.

I complete my cases in the morning and see consultations in the afternoon. Once we admit the patient, we take before photos. I draw where I will transfer the hairline to, then I get to work.

My job allows me to be creative because there is an element of finesse and design in the surgical planning. In addition, my job gives me autonomy, and a much better work-life balance.

But, to be honest, balance is still a work-in-progress. My current position makes everything easier because I arrive home at 7:30 p.m. or 8 p.m. Balance was easier when I had a live-in nanny. Now, my daughter is in daycare across from my office. This is convenient. I continue to work in a social life. When I figure out how to balance everything, I will let you know!

I feel my greatest accomplishment is my daughter. I never planned to have children. I was focused on my goals and establishing my career, so children were not a priority. I was 38 years old when I had my daughter, which is considered late, but she has been my greatest blessing.

Completing my surgical residency was another great accomplishment. Surgery training was difficult. There were times I wanted to give up, but I persisted. My father died when I was in medical school. His dying wish was to see me finish medical school and become a surgeon. Even though he was not here to see me through, I was still motivated to finish on his behalf. I could not let the sacrifices my family made (mom, I am looking at you), just fall by the wayside

As far as dealing with failure goes, I have a remarkable ability to block things out. I give myself a moment to mourn and be down about it and then I pick myself up and move on. I look at what caused my failure and make the necessary changes.

Lessons I would like to share with the up-and-coming young black woman who wants to be a physician are, it is especially important to read! Read all the time! It is important to take control of your education and development in surgical residency. Work hard to master your skills early on. It is important to have a strong support network, both at home and ideally someone at the hospital you can trust. Finding a mentor is key. I kept my mentors' phone numbers on speed-dial during my initial years as an attending. In medical school, don't take every student loan available just because you can, live simply. Try to live as simply as possible. Once in residency, start paying back the loans. Do this even if all you can afford is the interest-only payments. Learn about managing money early during residency. Protect your investment and find good disability insurance coverage early in your surgical training. Ideally you should do this before you develop any injuries or become pregnant because the premiums increase significantly for women thereafter.

My final words to all the ladies out there are, "I heard a wonderful quote by Suzy Kassem I love to recite to myself whenever I feel fear guiding my decisions. 'Doubt kills more dreams than failure ever will.' I hope this helps someone as much as it has helped me!"

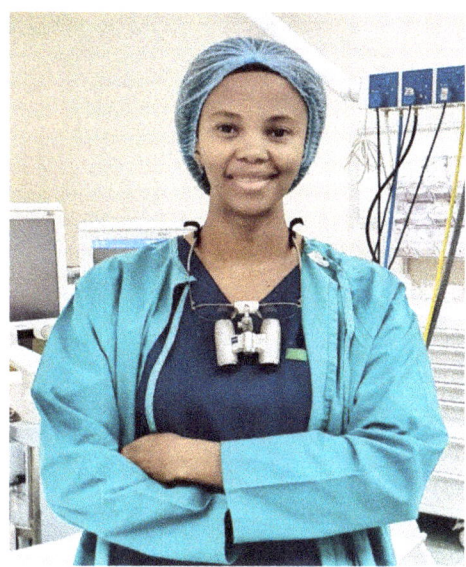

Dr. Elizabeth A. Xoagus-Makakole

    Dr. Elizabeth A. Xoagus-Makakole is a consultant plastic and reconstructive surgeon at Inkosi Albert Luthuli Hospital in Durban, South Africa. She earned her medical degree at the University of Cape Town in Cape Town, South Africa. She returned to her home country, Namibia, and completed her internship as she worked as a medical officer in general surgery. She returned to South Africa for her plastic surgery fellowship and became Namibia's first black female plastic surgeon. She is a fellow of the college of plastic surgeons of South Africa.

    Growing up, medicine is the only career Dr. Xoagus-Makakole dreamed of pursuing. As a child, she was motivated to pursue medicine when her mom was sick. Dr. Xoagus-Makakole felt helpless. Even when her mom was sick with a simple common cold it changed the atmosphere at home. Dr. Xoagus-Makakole did not like this atmosphere or seeing her mom sick. She thinks this subconsciously made her pursue her dream to become a medical doctor as a way to help.

    During her internship, her general surgery department head took it upon himself to convince her she should pursue a career in surgery. He believed she had the skills to do so. "You have good hands," he said. Dr. Xoagus-Makakole was the first female in a general surgery rotation performing general surgical procedures as a medical officer. This was not well received by many, including the nurses and some colleagues. Their reaction discouraged her from pursuing a career in surgery. She thanks God that her department head was insistent and pushed her to pursue surgery despite the opposition.

Dr. Xoagus-Makakole's first exposure to plastic surgery was when she was assigned to work with a group of visiting missionary plastic surgeons. There were no plastic surgery residents in her hospital at the time. During their two-week stay, the visiting team focused on reconstructive surgery. Dr. Xoagus-Makakole had the opportunity to observe a patient who was restored and regained lost function. This is why she fell in love with plastic surgery.

Her greatest challenge was facing and fighting discrimination. It was not easy, but she learned to be firm and knew what her rights were and are. She stood for what was right and is now well-respected in her field because she persevered.

Dr. Xoagus-Makakole attributes her strength and confidence to the fact that she is a born-again Christian. Her faith makes her confident because her confidence is in God and what He says about her in His Word. Her second source of confidence comes from her dearest mother who supported her and believed in her dream more than anyone else and who continues to encourage her. Dr. Xoagus-Makakole also draws support from the rest of her family and friends who believe in her and help keep her moving forward.

Dr. Xoagus-Makakole realized early on in her career path that she needed to prioritize things. Some things in life are of higher priority than others. Life requires one to be flexible and there are phases or periods where she prioritized some aspects of her life more than others.

It also means realizing and accepting she cannot do everything, and she must leave some things and defer others to another time. However, she feels it is crucial to remember that no important aspect of life should be neglected for too long.

Dr. Xoagus-Makakole considers her greatest accomplishments and proudest moments to be seeing her daughter following in her footsteps. Dr. Xoagus-Makakole does not mean her daughter talking about becoming a doctor but realizing she has set a good example for her daughter. Dr. Xoagus-Makakole sees her daughter dreaming big and believing in herself. This is reflected by her performance at school and her view and approach to academics.

When her daughter attended Dr. Xoagus-Makakole's master's graduation ceremony, she asked her mother what the highest qualification is that one could attain. When Dr. Xoagus-Makakole told her daughter, the highest qualification is a doctorate; her daughter promptly asked why she was not pursuing that! Dr. Xoagus-Makakole's daughter concluded her mother's not pursuing a doctorate was like dropping out of high school before completing her matriculation (final high school exams in southern Africa).

This was Dr. Xoagus-Makakole's proudest moment because she knows her daughter will achieve great things and she does not need to tell her daughter the importance of school, hard work, and striving for excellence. Her daughter knows these things. In other countries doctors have a master's degree as their highest degree and a doctorate is a PhD degree except for countries such as the USA and Philippines where a DO or MD degree is a doctorate.

On the flip side, Dr. Xoagus-Makakole finds how to deal with failure and complications a good question, but a difficult one. She does not think she will ever become immune to complications. She does not think anyone ever does! Dr. Xoagus-Makakole thinks we are all able to handle minor complications well, but major complications are more challenging. They affect every surgeon, otherwise, we would not have hearts.

Dr. Xoagus-Makakole feels that the sooner she realizes and accepts the reality that complications are part of the profession, the better it is for her and her patients. She allows herself to mourn the failure, but she does not dwell on it. She similarly celebrates the successful cases quietly and with humility. The fact that the successful cases are more the norm than are failures/complications also helps to deal with the sentiments around the failure/complications quickly and keeps her moving forward.

A typical day for Dr. Xoagus-Makakole depends on whether it is a clinic day or a theater (operating room) day. She starts with ward rounds at 8 a.m. on a clinic day, which last about two hours, followed by outpatient consults in the clinic.

Dr. Xoagus-Makakole works in clinic as with her team, the registrars (residents), and medical officers. They usually complete their work before 4 p.m. and have an academic program starting at 4 p.m., with a presentation prepared by a registrar or medical officer. This is followed by a journal club presentation from 5 to 6 p.m. prepared by a consultant.

She usually arrives home at about 7 p.m. on clinic days. Dr. Xoagus-Makakole serves supper, cleans up, then she tucks her daughter into bed. She either does administrative work at 10 p.m. before she goes to bed or just goes to bed when she is too tired to work more. If she does not get to her administrative the night before, she wakes early to complete it.

A typical theater day starts at 8 a.m. and ends around 5 p.m. most days but can continue until 6 or 7 p.m. depending on the complexity of the surgery she is performing.

Finally, Dr. Xoagus-Makakole would like to add, "First, you have to believe in yourself, otherwise, no one else will. Secondly, know you are enough just the way you are! Do not seek external validation. Master your craft and shine. Lastly, choose your battles wisely. Not everything is worth a fight."

CHAPTER TWENTY
Surgical Oncology

Surgical oncology is the branch of surgery applied to oncology (cancer); it focuses on the surgical management of tumors, especially cancerous tumors.

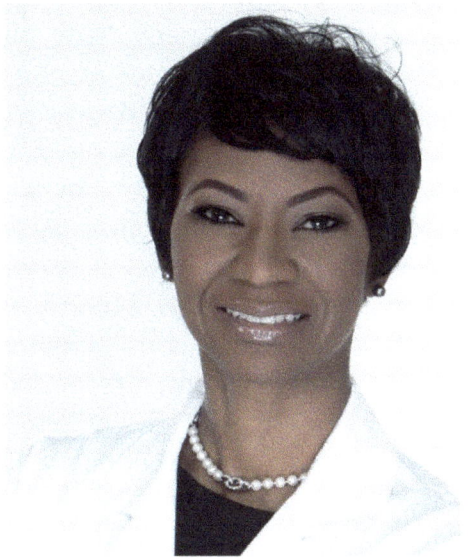

Dr. Lori Wilson

Dr. Lori Wilson is the division chief of surgical oncology at Howard University Hospital in Washington, D.C, and focuses on health disparities in underrepresented populations as well as breast, colorectal, and endocrine cancers.

She is also the program director of the general surgery residency at Howard University Hospital. As a graduate of Georgetown University School of Medicine in Washington, D.C., she completed her internship and residency in general surgery at Howard University Hospital. During this time, she was honored with the university's Chairman's Award, the Resident's Choice

Award from the department of surgery, and was inducted into Alpha Omega Alpha, Gamma Chapter, Medical Honor Society, along with other honors.

She completed her research fellowship at the University of Cincinnati in Ohio, with advanced coursework in cellular biology, molecular genetics, and bioethics. She finished her surgical oncology fellowship at the John Wayne Cancer Institute in Santa Monica, California, where she was honored as a chief administrative surgical oncology fellow.

Dr. Wilson's personal struggle with breast cancer is featured in the Ken Burns' PBS documentary, *Cancer: The Emperor of All Maladies,* based on the Pulitzer Prize-winning book by Dr. Siddhartha Mukherjee. She allowed cameras to film her surgery as she underwent a double mastectomy. She is a breast cancer survivor and works tirelessly to fight cancer daily.

This is Dr. Wilson's story.

My journey to become a surgeon began when I was seven years old. I always liked science and numbers in elementary school. I watched *MASH* and wanted to be like Hawkeye. He was the male surgeon who saved people and was good at what he did. It did not dawn on me that he did not look like me. I enjoyed watching the surgeons on *MASH* saving lives and using their abilities to help someone who was injured or sick. Even though this was fictitious, I loved how they immediately changed a patient's health.

When I was in elementary school. My parents purchased a set of encyclopedias that came with a medical encyclopedia as a bonus book. I liked the transparencies of the bones, muscles, and blood vessels. When I was in the 10th grade, I was selected to participate in a summer program focusing on cancer research. It was then that I decided I wanted to be a cancer surgeon.

My parents lived in the segregated south and waited until later in life to have me when more opportunities were available for black people. I was the first person in my family to finish college. My parents said if I worked hard, I could be whatever I wanted to be.

Now, I am a surgical oncologist, and I operate one or two days a week. I see patients in the clinic one or two days a week. I am also the program director for the general surgery residency managing 33 residents through their training. I also volunteer and provide more than 50 women with free mammography and clinical breast exams once a month.

My favorite part of my job is spending time with my patients and getting to know them as people. The operating room is my oasis. It is where I am most comfortable. Besides this, the best part of my job is being with my patients and knowing I have an impact.

My goal has always been making sure everyone has a fair and just opportunity and removing barriers that make outcomes different, whether these disadvantages are social, economic, or environmental. I spend my day partnering with women and men helping them understand the word cancer that has now become their diagnosis. I help them know what this diagnosis really means, what the treatment will do, and how they will look toward their future in a real and relevant way.

On a personal note, I was diagnosed with breast cancer in June 2013 when my son was 18 months old. After I stopped breastfeeding, one of my breasts did not decrease in size. This is abnormal, so I had a mammogram. I was devastated when I was told my diagnosis was breast cancer. I chose Johns Hopkins in Baltimore, Maryland, for treatment since I was well-known at Howard University Hospital where I worked. I just wanted to be a patient and Johns Hopkins was closer to my home.

On my first visit, I realized my medical oncologist was a woman I sat next to at a charity event months before. I was diagnosed with two types of invasive cancer in both breasts. One type of cancer was triple-negative, meaning the cancer cells did not have estrogen or progesterone receptors and did not make much of the protein called HER2.

HER2 cell receptors are special proteins found inside or on the surface of cells that receive signals from the bloodstream (hormones) that help the cells grow. So, this means triple-negative breast cancer does not respond to hormonal therapy medicine or medicines that target HER2 protein receptors because these hormone receptors are not present on the cells. This is the most aggressive breast cancer and has the worst prognosis for survival. I underwent 16 treatments of chemotherapy followed by a double mastectomy with immediate reconstruction. I also received 30 treatments of radiation to my chest wall and hormonal therapy. I am a survivor.

I think as a doctor I was a fairly good patient. During my last year of training as a surgical resident, my mother was diagnosed with lung cancer and I spent that year caring for her and experiencing cancer as a caregiver. My mother wanted to stay at home during the end of her life and this taught me about humility and letting go and allowing people to care for you.

I learned from her is that it is ok to let people who love and care about you take care of you when you really need it and are vulnerable. If I had not experienced this, I would probably not have been a good patient. But I was determined to let go and not direct my care.

I asked my doctors to treat me as they would any other patient and explain everything to me the way they would explain things to their regular patients. I was fortunate to have the resources I have. I had my surgery at Cedar Sinai in Los Angeles, California, by my mentor Dr. Armando Giuliano, who trained me thirteen years prior. Being a patient was a humbling experience.

Dr. Giuliano shared, "We all loved Lori when she was a surgical oncology fellow. She was very hardworking, very smart, fun to be with, completely reliable, and very inquisitive. She had a spark. I knew she would do something with her life and career!"

CHAPTER TWENTY-ONE
Oral and Maxillofacial Surgery

Oral and maxillofacial surgeons are trained to recognize and treat a wide spectrum of diseases, injuries and defects in the head, neck, face, jaw, and the hard and soft tissues of the oral and maxillofacial region. They are also trained to administer anesthesia and provide care in an office setting. They treat problems such as the extraction of wisdom teeth, misaligned jaws, tumors and cysts of the jaw and mouth, and to perform dental implant surgery. Oral and maxillofacial surgery is a surgical specialty recognized by the American College of Surgeons and is one of nine dental specialties recognized by the American Dental Association, the Royal College of Dentists of Canada, and the Royal Australasian College of Dental Surgeons.

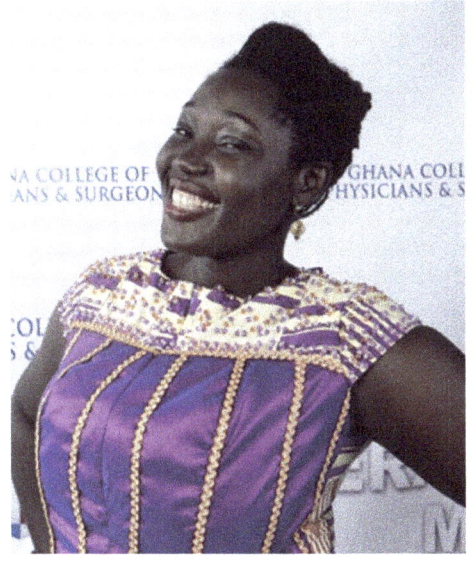

Dr. Sandra Oyakhilome

Dr. Sandra Oyakhilome is the head of dental and oral maxillofacial surgery (OMFS) at Cape Coast Teaching Hospital in Ghana, Africa. She completed her bachelor's degree in medical sciences at the University of Ghana in Africa. She earned a Bachelor of Dental Surgery (BDS) at the University of Ghana Dental School. She worked as a house-officer for two years at Korlebu Teaching Hospital & Ridge Regional Hospital, and as a medical officer at Cape Coast Teaching Hospital in Ghana.

Dr. Oyakhilome was admitted to the Ghana College of Physicians and Surgeons and completed her residency training in oral maxillofacial surgery at Komfo Anoyke Teaching Hospital in Ghana to become a member of the Ghana College of Surgeons. She emerged as the first female Ghanaian-trained oral and maxillofacial surgeon in the country. She became the second female maxillofacial surgeon in the county, the first female maxillofacial surgeon was foreign-trained Professor Grace Parkins. She returned to Cape Coast Teaching Hospital after residency as a specialist. She is married with one child.

Dr. Oyakhilome chose dentistry because she loves to create things with her hands and put smiles on people's faces. Dentistry offers the ability to restore healthy smiles, OMFS because it extends beyond the mouth and also focuses on the face.

She practices in a government teaching hospital healthcare facility. This requires a great deal of mental and physical strength along with endless patience because of the doctor-to-patient ratio. Currently, there is one doctor to 4,000 people. There is a tremendous amount of skill required to work with limited resources and still save lives and have a life as a physician.

Currently, Dr. Oyakhilome is the acting head of her dental and OMFS department, so a typical day is a mixture of management duties as well as clinical and supervisory duties. She starts her day with her morning routine. She arrives on the patient wards to review patients admitted overnight.

She also sees patients in the accident and emergency department and discusses these patients with her team and colleagues. They make plans for patients to be discharged to home or be admitted to the ward.

Each day, Dr. Oyakhilome heads to the Dental/OMFS outpatient department (clinic) to evaluate patients. In clinic, she consults with patients and does minor surgeries. She trains and supervises doctors in training. Some days she is in the theater (operating room) doing major operations. At the end of the day, she passes through the wards to check on post-operative patients before heading home. Dr. Oyakhilome also attends meetings throughout the day. She frequently checks in with the emergency department to make sure there are no patients that need her attention before heading home. She keeps her phone close in case there are emergencies.

Dr. Oyakhilome considers her greatest accomplishment to be being the youngest first female Ghanaian-trained oral and maxillofacial surgeon to become a member of the Ghana College of Surgeons in 2018 and her proudest moment the day she became a mother.

When discussing balance, Dr. Oyakhilome claims that anyone working in a demanding profession, surgery or otherwise, who tells you that work-life balance is possible, is conning you. Life will never be in perfect balance. You must find a way to integrate all aspects of your life and make sure to constantly reevaluate, so you do not neglect an area in your life.

There is no such thing as a perfect parent, surgeon, or wife. You must be gentle with yourself and understand there is no such thing as balance.

She believes life is about sacrifice and the only things to balance are rest and recovery. After all, on the last day, God rested. The rest of the days you should be creating and focusing on your vision, passion, and goals. You should be growing. So, weekends are the days she spends resting and recovering. Dr. Oyakhilome shuffles between staying at home, going on outings with her family and friends, and fellowshipping with other Christians.

Dr. Oyakhilome feels that having lived in West Africa all her life, being black has never been an issue. She is blessed to be in an environment that supports women and respect is conferred once you are a doctor, whether male or female.

Her greatest challenge as a dentist is having people appreciate the importance of oral health as part of general health and not waiting until there is pain before they seek dental care. Public oral health education and access to oral healthcare services is a huge challenge.

Dr. Oyakhilome's encouraging and kind words for each reader are, "Have a long-term vision for your career and have faith in God to see you through. Take time to develop a career plan and set timelines. Be bold and just do it. Ask questions. Do not listen to people who have the, "It can't be done," mindset. Be persistent. Yes. We. Can."

"What could we accomplish if we knew we could not fail?"
— Eleanor Roosevelt

CHAPTER TWENTY-TWO
Doctors in Surgical Training

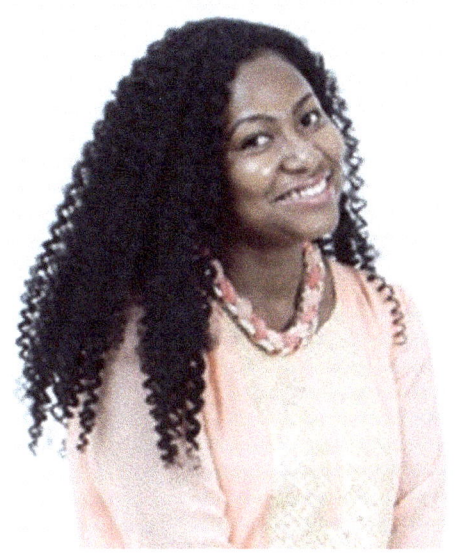

Dr. Josephine Kusano

Dr. Josephine Kusano is a junior registrar (resident) in the department of urology at United Bulawayo Hospitals in Zimbabwe, Africa. She completed her medical school training at Wenzhou Medical College in Wenzhou, Zhejiang, China, and is completing her surgical training in Zimbabwe.

This is her journey from Ghana to China to Zimbabwe.

I was born and raised in Ghana, Africa. My passion to pursue medicine goes as far back as my primary school days in Ghana. I know most people think it is a cliche, but some doctors are inspired at a young age. I always thought of myself becoming a doctor when I grew up and I loved assisting our school nurse with wound care. I did not know what I was doing, but it made me feel good making my classmates think I could fix them. I made sure to work hard in school and I excelled scholastically. I told myself that one day I would be a doctor and all my classmates would come to me for care.

In junior high school, I attended a renowned private school in the capital city Accra in Ghana, Africa, and there were a few classmates who called me, "Miss Know-it-All." I remember my principal advised me to separate myself from these classmates to strengthen myself and excel.

These years were difficult because I had few friends and many enemies, but it never diminished my self-confidence. I told myself that if my parents, principal, and few friends saw something great in me, then I could be so much more than I could imagine.

When I was a senior in high school, I succumbed to a wave of peer pressure, a bit of truancy, and some regression in my academics. My mother threatened to pull me from the science program and move me to the home economics program. I cried and promised to do better. Luckily, my beloved father came to my rescue and gave me another chance to remain in the science program. He realized how much I loved learning science.

From then on, I worked extremely hard, but it was not enough to excel on my final national exams. Because I did not do as well as I needed to on my national exams, I decided to pursue law. I watched many television crime series and read legal thrillers, so I thought it would be a great career. I lost hope of being accepted into medical school because of my poor performance but thought I could excel as a lawyer.

My father never gave up on my going to medical school. He invited a friend who was a neurosurgeon to talk to me and encourage me to not give up. With this reassurance, I applied to medical school and was accepted into one of the medical universities in Ghana. I was excited but also afraid of the difficulties of a medical education. I heard stories about it being exceedingly difficult, and about some students succumbing to the pressures and committing suicide or quitting. I wondered if I was good enough to complete medical school.

As fate would have it, my mother decided she did not want

me to complete my medical training in Ghana, where I would be exposed to my friends and peer pressure. She gave me the choice of applying to the University of Maryland in the U.S. to pursue a non-medical, non-legal undergraduate course of study or applying to the Wenzhou Medical University in China to pursue a medical degree. I chose China and this jump-started my journey to become a doctor.

Medical school was a roller coaster. I met my husband, a Zimbabwean young man also pursuing a medical degree. When we met, he became my best friend. We became each other's support system and helped one another stay focused on our studies. We joked that I was the medical physician and he was the surgeon in our study group.

I remember the dread I felt when I was the second assistant for a plastic surgery case. The patient was an adorable female toddler who needed her bilateral cleft lip repaired. A cleft lip is a birth defect that results in an opening or split in the upper lip and interferes with feeding.

When I started medical school, I considered medicine rather than surgery and intentionally avoided assisting in surgical procedures. However, this cleft lip operation was the turning point in my career.

Anxiously, I assisted by cutting the sutures at just the right length and exerting sufficient traction with the skin hooks. I avoided anything that might upset the surgeon operating because it could have resulted in a scolding. But, when I saw that child smile for the first time after we removed the bandages, I knew surgery was what I wanted to do for the rest of my life.

When I was an intern rotating in the surgical department at one of the main referral hospitals in Harare, the capital of Zimbabwe, I was stressed. After a traumatizing three months of general surgery, I was scared and petrified. I felt traumatized because general surgeons can be difficult to work with and training is intense. I spent long hours standing in the operating room dealing with distressing injuries and assisting with complicated surgeries.

I rotated on the maxillofacial surgery service and, even though they were more accommodating and patient than the general surgeons, I resisted the urge to develop an interest in surgery.

Interns are required to attend maxillofacial, dental, and plastic surgery clinics three times a week. I developed an interest in clinic patients because I was able to see post-operative patients. This was great because my consultant always took before photos, and when the patients came for their follow-up clinic visit, we took the after photos. The transformation was amazing.

Every day I told myself I would be the first doctor in my family when I returned home, work at the hospital of my dreams in Accra, and walk around wearing my white coat with a big smile. I imagined my mum looking at me, a successful doctor, and telling my dad how he had made the right decision allowing me to complete my science program in senior high school when she wanted me to switch to home economics.

I excelled in medical school until one month before my final exams. I was only weeks from graduation when my father died from bronchogenic carcinoma. I was devastated and I almost quit medical school out of anger and grief. I thought I was going to lose my mind. It was a dark time in my life. My husband and close friends rallied around me and helped me deal with my grief. I was able to study for my exams and passed. I wished my dad could have been here to see me become the great person he hoped me to be.

My husband and I moved to his home, Zimbabwe, and I began my internship at Harare Central Hospital. This was when I discovered my hidden love for surgery.

Everyone asked, "Why not pursue plastic surgery since this was the surgical discipline that originally captivated me?" After my internship, I accepted a job in Bulawayo as a hospital medical officer. This was the only available post (position) at the time. When I worked in the urology department, I developed a sudden interest in it. I found a great mentor who has been a great guide and helped me realize that even though urology is a male-dominated specialty in Zimbabwe, what matters most are my skills and not my gender. He said if I have a passion for urology, then I should do it.

Some days are challenging, and some are fulfilling. This is what keeps me going and makes me enjoy my career. With great support from my mother, my husband, and my children, I feel I can conquer all the obstacles I face. When I get home, I love turning some of my experiences at work into fictional bedtime stories. My children love my stories! I am glad to say I have motivated my two older children to aspire to be doctors in the future.

I have three children. My oldest is a 12-year-old girl. She is my husband's biological child, but I have raised her since my husband and I met. She is mine. We also have two younger boys, a five-year-old and a seven-month-old. It has not been easy juggling work, family, and children. Sometimes I feel I am about to collapse from fatigue and exhaustion. I am someone who likes to put my whole heart and effort into accomplishing things I set my mind to do.

Urology training is difficult and terribly busy. I am training at a major referral hospital and there are many patients coming to our facility. Unfortunately, with the doctors in training strike, there are fewer of us to get the work done. Because of the strikes, my consult and I are on call every day. I rely on my support system, especially when I am working so many hours.

Sometimes, my children are disappointed when I leave them with their aunty who cares for them while I work. She is a wonderful lady and I am grateful for her help. On any free day, I make sure I cook our meals and bake with my daughter and sometimes take her for a girls' outing. Other times, my husband and I take all the children for a family outing or a short trip.

Luckily, my husband wants me to become a urologist as much as I do. He encourages me to fill my case logbook and to study urology. He asked one of his friends at the hospital records department to gather all the necessary data for my dissertation. My husband assists with some chores and sometimes visits me at work for lunch.

What keeps me going is knowing I make my family proud of me and also the sense of personal satisfaction when I see my patients grateful for the help I give them.

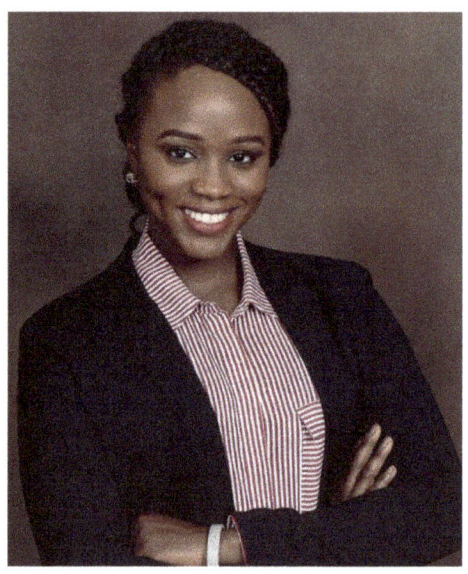

Odinachi Moghalu Schulle

Dr. Odinachi Moghalu Schulle received her bachelor's degree in biomedical engineering from Baylor University in Waco, Texas. She has a master's in biomedical science from Touro College of Osteopathic Medicine, New York, New York, where she also received her Doctor of Osteopathic Medicine degree.

She completed an internship in general surgery at New York Presbyterian Queens Hospital in Flushing, New York. She is currently a post-doctoral research fellow at the University of Utah, School of Medicine in Salt Lake City, Utah, in the department of surgery, urology division.

Dr. Moghalu Schulle wanted to become a doctor since she was three years old. She does not recall any specific events that led her to this decision, however, after high school, she chose to pursue mathematics and physics. This led her to earn a degree in engineering.

Since she did not have a reason why she chose medicine, Dr. Moghalu Schulle wanted to make sure this decision was hers, not something her parents subconsciously instilled in her. So, rather than go straight into medical school after high school, how it is done in England where she lived at the time, she made the decision to pursue engineering. She chose biomedical engineering.

During her undergraduate studies, she realized she was interested in medicine, but at the same time, she did not want to let go of her engineering background. Dr. Moghalu Schulle's interest went from considering a career in medicine to finding how she would be able to merge her deep interest in engineering and human physiology.

During her third-year clinical rotation in medical school, she experienced the greatest joy during her surgery clinical rotations. When she was in the operating room (OR), in a place of controlled chaos, she had an overwhelming feeling of satisfaction. It was the most strenuous and tasking rotation, but it was the one rotation where she felt like she never wanted to leave the hospital.

Dr. Moghalu Schulle is currently a post-doctoral research fellow at the University of Utah in the department of surgery, urology division. She completed her general surgery internship.

A typical day as an intern was quite different from a typical day Dr. Moghalu Schulle now has as a research fellow. As an intern, her day started at 3:30 a.m. when her alarm went off and she prepared herself for work. She typically tried to be out of her apartment between 5:15 and 5:30 a.m. so she was at work no later than 5:45 a.m. On days she took sign-out (report to continue care) from the person who was on night float, she arrived by 5:30 a.m. to allow time to receive the sign-out, transfer the on-call phone, and not have to rush through the details.

General sign-out with the entire department usually started at 6 a.m., and they tried to be finished no later than 6:30 a.m. for team morning rounds. This is where they walked around and evaluated each patient on their list. Patients were in the emergency department, the patient units, and the intensive care unit.

Depending on the team she was on, Dr. Moghalu Schulle either headed to morning conference with the attending on call or could be found at her workstation at work on orders, notes, discharges, and patient care plans. When on day-call, she was not assigned OR cases or clinic time unless they were short-staffed on residents. If she was not on day-call, she headed to the operating room to learn to operate while assisting with cases.

Dr. Moghalu Schulle asserts graduating medical school, despite health issues that threatened her medical school journey, is the greatest accomplishment in her life so far. She is also proud of her determination and zeal.

Now, she is involved in an unpaid research position. This is difficult considering she could have stayed in general surgery, a specialty for which she has no deep passion. Dr. Moghalu Schulle made this difficult choice to take an unpaid research position hoping her portfolio will become stronger. This is so she can successfully apply to a specialty she is genuinely interested in, urology.

Dr. Moghalu Schulle feels her greatest challenge has been finding mentors who are black female urologists.

She has received so much good advice from people, but one bit of advice she finds herself going back to time and time again is, "You cannot be a doctor if you are dead." Her mum first said this to her when she was in high school. Her mum had been with her all her life, paying close attention to how zealously Dr. Moghalu Schulle extended herself to achieve success. Many times, this was to the detriment to her health. That day in high school, her mum finally had enough and insisted she drop everything and forced her to take time to rest.

Dr. Moghalu Schulle never took her mum seriously until she became extremely ill while in medical school and was almost forced to take a leave of absence. Her mum's words rang in her ears. They are true. Dr. Moghalu Schulle can only be a successful doctor if she is in the best health. She must prioritize her own health to best serve her patients.

Dr. Moghalu Schulle has had a few failures in her life, more like many, but has found that failure can either propel you or suffocate you. She finds when she experiences failure, she sits and cries. She cries out and expresses her feelings. She prays and then develops a strategy for how to get back up from that place. Dr. Moghalu Schulle looks at what she could have done differently and tries to separate things she can change from things she cannot change. For the things she can change, she works on these things to see how or where she can improve.

Dr. Moghalu Schulle considers herself an introvert and a recluse, so after a busy day or busy season, coming home and catching up on some of her favorite television shows or working out helps with stress. This for her is balance.

There are several lessons Dr. Moghalu Schulle would like to share. As a pre-medical student, she wishes someone had told her she did not have to rush to take the medical college admission test (MCAT) to fit a particular schedule.

She wishes the importance of seeking a mentor was emphasized. Dr. Moghalu Schulle also wishes she knew she could have taken time from medical school to pursue research in a specialty she was interested in. This is especially important since she had no research background before medical school.

Dr. Moghalu Schulle's lesson learned as an intern was people have more confidence in you if you have confidence in yourself. She is not talking about blind confidence or arrogance but walking into a room with the authority that earned her her place there. Being the only black female during her intern year, she felt like an impostor and several seniors took advantage of this. You must realize you earned that spot just like every other intern there, so act like it. Stay humble but be confident.

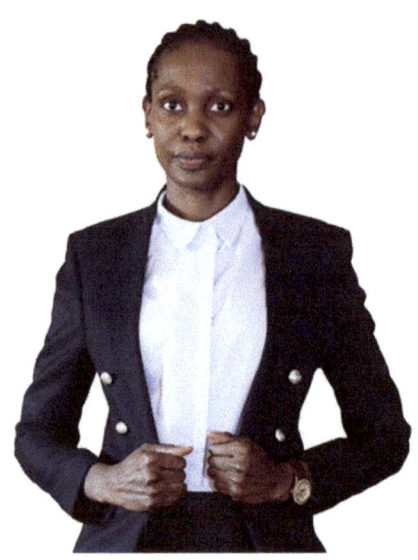

Dr. Weludo Ngwisanyi

Dr. Weludo Ngwisanyi is a general surgery registrar (resident) at Chris Hani Baragwanath Hospital, University of the Witwatersrand, South Africa. She completed her medical school education at the University of West Indies in Kingston, Jamaica.

This is her journey from Botswana to Jamaica to South Africa.

On one Friday night, as I left the casualty area (emergency department), I heard my junior's voice echoing through the entire casualty area. "RESUS," she screamed. This means resuscitation. We walked quickly toward her. The nursing sisters (nurses) know what this means and came running with their resuscitation trolley. Everyone jumped into action and assumed their specific roles.

As a resident, I was the team leader when my consultant was not present. Our patient was a young lady stabbed in the chest during a robbery and she was being resuscitated. The team worked diligently to save her. They gave her blood transfusions, fluid drips, medications, oxygen, and as the team leader, I made the decision to operate. I felt this was necessary to save her life.

We ran through the hospital corridors to the theater (operating room) and moved her to the operating table within minutes. The amazing theater team understood the urgency and within minutes my consultant and I opened her chest. We found that her heart was stabbed. We took our time and carefully and skillfully repaired the injured tissue. She lived and was discharged to her home within a few days! On days like this, I realize how fragile life is, how every minute matters, and the importance of timely decision making. If you miss it or if you make wrong decisions, patients die.

I am a 31-year-old female medical doctor from Botswana, Africa. I completed my medical training in Jamaica in 2014 and after earning my medical degree, I returned to Botswana to work as a medical doctor.

In January 2018, I entered the University of the Witwatersrand, South Africa, as a self-sponsored trainee in general surgery. This is a five-year training program. I decided to be brave and sponsor myself because the government of Botswana did not have an allocated budget to sponsor doctors for post-graduate studies.

From a young age, I knew I wanted to be a medical doctor. I am the third of five children. We were raised by our single mother on a meager salary. To me, my mother remains a true reflection of the strength of a woman. Therefore, working hard has always been something our mother instilled in us. I partly attribute my mother's great qualities to her family, who would occasionally help her care for us.

My childhood was typical for where I grew up. In order to attend junior secondary school, I walked 14 kilometers to and from school each day. Even after walking this distance, I was expected to help with daily chores in the house in addition to finishing my homework. My chores included cleaning the kitchen and looking after my baby brothers. I did not consider helping with chores work. I assumed this was part of the responsibilities of every girl child.

I spent my senior secondary school years at a boarding

school. I left the only comfort I knew – my mother's house. When I met fellow students from wealthy families, I realized I was from a poor economic background.

A small group of us from poor families depended on the school for food, but the children from wealthy families had an abundant supply. After evening studies, our colleagues from rich families ate the food they brought from home while we poor students slipped under our blankets. We were ashamed and hoped our stomachs did not grumble. Despite these challenges, I was determined to become a doctor.

For me, it has always been about working hard and working smart. It never occurred to me I was intelligent. All I knew was I needed to work hard to pass exams. Like any other boarding school, the curfews were enforced, and I felt the evening study time was inadequate.

Against all odds, I successfully completed my senior secondary school with excellent grades and through my government sponsorship, I found myself in Jamaica at the University of West Indies.

You would believe it would have gotten better, but this is not so. Medical school was difficult, and it took more effort to keep good grades and learn. My secret strategy was being part of a study group. I do not believe one person can know everything. Sharing knowledge and teamwork were what helped me through the rivers and valleys. Being far from my family and missing home was one of the challenges I had to overcome daily, but I kept my eyes fixed on the prize. Time sure does fly when you are busy!

When I completed medical school five years later, I returned home to Botswana. I was excited to be reunited with my family and serve the people of Mamaland. After studying medicine for five years, you would think this fully prepared me for the medical fraternity and all its challenges, but this was not true. I found myself saying, "I am not ready for this," half the time during my internship year.

One of the greatest challenges I faced, and still face, is having to deliver bad news to patients and families. This is even more difficult when a sudden or unexpected death occurs. Despite staring death in the face each day, it does not get easier. I guess this is because we are all still human at the end of the day.

Enduring long working hours, swollen feet, fighting sleep, and exhaustion, I finished my internship year. I progressed to junior medical officer. But, because Botswana, like other African countries, has challenges related to the shortage of doctors, especially specialists, this inspired me to focus on general surgery.

This is how I came to one of the busiest trauma centers in the world, the Chris Hani Baragwanath Hospital in South Africa. On many occasions, I find myself and fellow doctors working late, running casualty (emergencies) alone or with only two doctors on busy days. Patients must wait long hours. Though this is exhausting, it is fulfilling work if you are passionate about serving people this way.

Currently, God willing, I will complete my surgery specialty training in three years and return to Mamaland (Botswana) to serve my people – as a qualified surgeon.

Surgery training in South Africa is one of the most intense programs. It is filled with a wide range of illnesses since it is one of the largest hospitals in Africa. Chris Hani Baragwanath Hospital has more than 3,000 beds. The trauma surgery department is such a busy place it makes you think there is a war underway. The experience has been amazing with a great deal of operating time and teaching. Currently, I am working on my research study, which I hope to have published in a year.

Training in general surgery is not without its challenges. I feel it is a male-dominated specialty. So, it goes with the territory that a young female must work extra hard to show she is capable. I find myself on ward rounds with male surgeons I feel have huge egos.

As a resident, you are expected to know your patients thoroughly, operate on them, run the clinic, make academic presentations, and supervise and teach junior doctors as well as medical students. Additionally, I must work 24-hour call duty, which sometimes turns into 30-hour call duty, and work on my research. We have weekends off to recover and visit with family.

As an African woman, it is challenging to pursue a career and be a homemaker, find a partner, get married, and have children, as per societal expectations. You learn that even your family is not impressed with your choices when they feel other aspects of life are being delayed, because you are expected to focus on homemaking. When I think of the long working hours, the sacrifices, and the exhaustion, I know it will eventually pay off.

If there is any advice, I would give myself at each stage of life, it would be to remain focused and work hard. Also, never forget where you come from. The hardships in life make us who we are. We become strong young women because of where we come from. Always remember to stay grounded. Do not let anyone tell you what you can or cannot do. Never limit yourself. Spread your wings and fly like a butterfly, young girl. There are thousands of opportunities in the world, even beyond your current environment. Never be afraid to dream big dreams. Be ambitious and go all out. It is not easy, but it can be done. Remember everything happens for a reason. There is a God up there watching. You will overcome every obstacle. Never give up. Never quit! It is all worth it.

"You may not always have a comfortable life and you will not always be able to solve all of the world's problems at once but don't ever underestimate the importance you can have because history has shown us that courage can be contagious and hope can take on a life of its own." – Michelle Obama

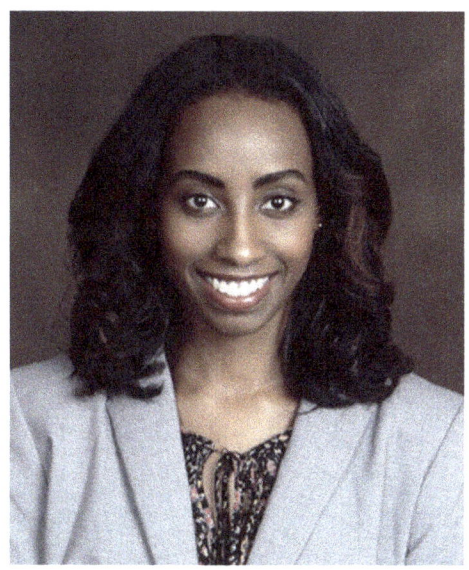

Dr. Ivy Godana

Dr. Ivy Godana is a general surgery resident at McLaren Greater Lansing, Michigan State University in East Lansing, Michigan. She earned her bachelor's degree from Baylor University in Waco, Texas, and a master's in clinical sciences from Boston University School of Medicine, Boston, Massachusetts. She completed her Doctor of Osteopathic Medicine from A.T. Still University of Health Sciences in Mesa, Arizona.

This is Dr. Ivy Godana's story in her words.

Mine has not been a straightforward journey. It seems many people know they want to be doctors from a young age. This was not so for me! I was born and raised in Kenya. I am half Kenyan and half Ethiopian.

We moved to Dallas, Texas, USA, when I was 10 years old. My parents were keen to make certain we understood the importance of education. My father said, "You are here to accomplish something, and you have to take advantage of the opportunity." Therefore, school was a priority for us.

When I was in high school, I realized I liked biology and I also liked health science classes. I loved English classes and read extensively, so my mom encouraged me to consider a career in medicine. I did not think I was smart enough or good enough to be a physician. However, I did have the courage to pursue the dream of medicine because I learned early on that courage is not the absence of fear but the doing despite the fear.

For me, high school was divided into two segments. During my first two years, I was not serious about school. I was satisfied with B's and did not push myself. My dad died when I was in the middle of high school. This was a difficult time, but it resulted in a huge shift in the way I approached life.

My dad wanted us to work hard and do well. He was an attorney and told my mom, my sisters, and me that education is the key to the future. Knowledge is power. This stuck with me, even till today. When I look back at my high school self, I would say, "You are having fun, but remember the important things in life. Keep going. You are doing well. You'll be fine."

When I took the SAT, I told God I wanted to go to Baylor for my undergraduate education and by God's grace, I did well on the SAT and was accepted into my number one choice, Baylor. My mother was excited for me. I was exposed to many things and had many opportunities there. I learned about global medicine and epidemiology. I had fantastic professors and it was a pre-medicine (pre-med) driven school. I became immersed in the pre-med world and knew for sure I wanted to be a physician.

I met one of my mentors in college, Dr. Baker. To my surprise, he coordinated an annual medical mission trip to Kenya, my own home country. The trip was to Western Kenya, so when I joined him it was as though I had come full circle. It was an amazing opportunity to see and feel what it is like to be a healthcare provider in my homeland.

I am proud of my heritage and because I grew up in Kenya, I am more familiar with this culture. Now, I am learning much more about my Ethiopian heritage. It was wonderful to be home and reconnect with everyone. I was grateful.

Being accepted to medical school was not easy because my MCAT score was not the best and my GPA was average compared to others applying. I knew I needed to do something to stand out. What followed was a life lesson in rejection. I applied to medical school after college and it was a resounding rejection from everywhere. I was extremely disappointed and sank into a depression.

I had this huge dream and I worked hard, but the doors kept closing in my face. You begin to think your dream is never going to happen. My mother encouraged me to keep believing and continue with my education, so I enrolled in a master's program at Boston University. After finishing my master's degree, I applied to medical school again. Guess what? Resounding rejection again!

Yes, it was difficult, but there is one thing I realized, in hindsight, I was usually a late applicant. This was a problem because most medical schools filled their seats by the time I applied. Just because there is a deadline does not mean you should wait until that deadline.

Be organized and get your application in early! I told myself, "You have to try again. There is no reason why you can't try again." I was more afraid of missing an opportunity than failing. So, I submitted my application early the next round.

I remember sitting in our living room and working hard on my secondary applications to medical school listing all the reasons I was good enough and would make a great physician. That cycle, I received many rejections, but guess what? I was granted one interview. One. One interview at A.T. Still in Arizona!

All I needed was one medical school to give me a chance. My first choice for medical school was the George Washington University because I wanted to live in Washington, D.C., and they had a well-known global medicine program. Later, by God's providence, an opportunity presented itself and I was able to complete my clinical years in Washington, D.C.

I cried tears of joy when I was accepted into medical school. I knew then that my dream was possible. I love reading. One of my favorite writers is Rumi. There is a quote where he asks, "Why have I received only this?" A voice replied, "Only this will lead you to that." I did not need a slew of choices. Sometimes God gives you exactly and only what you need. Revelation 3:7 says, "To the angel of the church in Philadelphia write: These are the words of Him Who is Holy and True, Who holds the key of David. What He opens, no one can shut, and what He shuts, no one can open."

When I sent my deposit to reserve my position, I felt this was something God had given me. It has not been an easy road. I cried many times thinking it was over. Now, I marvel as I look back on my journey to becoming who I am today. I learned that your strength is in your perseverance. It is not in the things you have been successful in; it is in the many times where you fall and you decide, I'd rather get back up and fall again than not try at all. God is good!

It is because of all these experiences that I am better prepared for surgical residency. I didn't always realize it, but those moments when I had to pull every ounce of strength from within to get back up, were character building. One of the things that helps is this little poem by a little girl from Malawi. It says, "Little by little we go." A friend of mine sent it to me and I wrote it out. Training was difficult, the hours are long, and the stakes are extremely high. I am learning to take one step at a time, even if it is one little step every day until I achieve my goal.

When I look back and compare it with residency, medical school was not so bad. But at that moment, it seemed difficult. In medical school, you learn a great deal of information, but you also learn much about yourself. You learn how you deal with stress and how you respond to stress. I also learned much about time management. I learned about the importance of taking care of myself first. You must be strong in mind, body, and spirit to be productive, efficient, and successful.

I had great professors. If your mind and heart are open to receiving, you are going to receive the information. What worked for me was finding a study group and balancing studying with people and studying alone. Alone, because you are a physician alone. You are not going to be a physician with other people. You must determine what works for you because there is a great deal of information. The first two years are preparation for the next step. Learn to study well in college, so you develop the good study skills needed in medical school.

My clinical years were fun because I put what I was learning into practice. You are not writing real orders or doing real notes, but you are learning how the system works and the art of medicine.

I had an opportunity to rotate through Howard University in Washington, D.C, and it was so nice to be around people who looked like me. I developed relationships with other students and residents and was encouraged and inspired by many amazing residents and attendings. I had such a great time.

I would tell myself in those first few years, "Do not worry about the fun stuff. It will come later. Focus on the important things." In medical school, I would say, "Keep going. You are doing well. Everything is going to come together."

What I would like to leave every black girl or young lady with a dream of becoming a doctor is, "I want to say to those little girls to have huge dreams; no matter what your circumstances, you have a purpose. You belong here just as much as everyone else and you matter. Whatever dreams you have, it is like the valid words Lupita Nyong'o said, 'The world does not belong to a select few, it belongs to us all. Our greatest hindrances are our minds. If you say you are going to do something and you consistently put in the work and do your best, you will be rewarded."

"The future rewards those who press on. I don't have time to feel sorry for myself. I don't have time to complain. I'm going to press on."
– Barack Obama

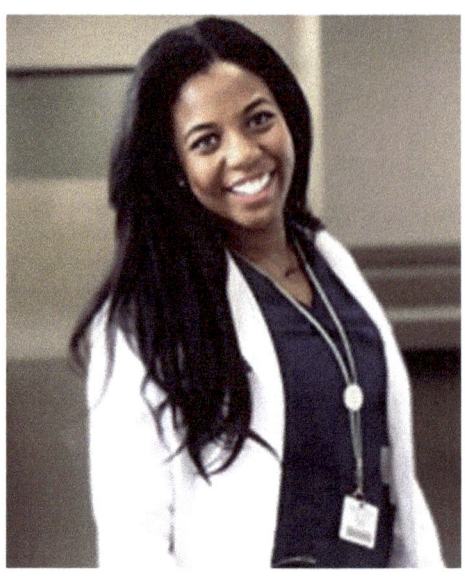

Dr. Amber Hardeman

Dr. Amber Hardeman is a surgical intern at the University of Mississippi Medical Center, Jackson, Mississippi. She earned her Bachelor of Arts degree in Spanish language and literature from Vanderbilt University in Nashville, Tennessee, and her master of public health from the University of Alabama in Birmingham. She earned a combined doctor of medicine and master of business administration from Tulane University School of Medicine and Tulane University A.A. Freeman School of Business, New Orleans, Louisiana.

This is Dr. Hardeman's story in her words.

I grew up as a military child. My parents were both in the Navy and, unlike most children, I moved from place to place. Moving was not an issue for me, but rather another adventure that optimized sharing experiences with others. I lived in many different states from California to Colorado to Texas, and other countries such as Japan and Australia. Every time I enrolled in a new school, I experienced a new culture, new friends, and new ideas. Another cornerstone growing up was golf. I was a member of the First Tee and not only played in the program, but I also participated as a mentor and eventual program director. I played in numerous tournaments on the Junior PGA tour, spoke at national PGA events, created PGA commercials, taught children to play golf, and eventually was recruited to play golf in college.

Growing up, I always knew I wanted to be a doctor because of my interest in science. As I became older, my passion for people solidified my career decision. I chose medicine because it empowers me to help people in a way that is not possible in any other field. Being a doctor is one of the most meaningful ways to positively contribute to society.

I chose surgery because there is a unique bond between a patient and a surgeon. The patient allows the surgeon to do something life-altering. The surgeon has the responsibility of someone's life in his or her hands. Complications are real, but positive outcomes and life satisfaction are exponential.

I believe healthcare is a right, not a privilege. I want to work in underserved communities as part of my mission to provide quality care. My desire to treat the patient rather than just the disease encouraged me to pursue an MD/MBA degree in addition to my MPH. I know that in addition to treating patients, medicine also involves understanding population-based health concerns, navigating the world of the healthcare business, and properly executing scientific knowledge to heal people.

As a bilingual black female, I have experienced firsthand treating patients who confide in me due to language and/or cultural barriers in care. I am dedicated to helping families have access to adequate healing support and diminishing disparities with adverse effects on public health.

My undergraduate experience was non-traditional. I was recruited for golf and accepted to Dartmouth College in Hanover, New Hampshire, in its early decision program. Over the course of the year, I realized I was not happy and searched for somewhere else to pursue my interests. I transferred to Vanderbilt University in Nashville, Tennessee, where I thrived.

I continued to play golf. I also dove deep into serving the

Nashville community as a member of the student government Community Service Board. I became a Spanish interpreter at the Vanderbilt University Medical Center. After school hours, I worked at the Vanderbilt Childcare Center. Also, I was on the boards for other clubs including the Global Health Committee and the Vanderbilt chapter of the NAACP. My goals in college were to study hard but still have fun.

I studied in Spain while working on my Spanish honor's thesis. I also traveled abroad for community service projects in Costa Rica and Guatemala. I tried to make the best of my time, remain well rounded, yet also adequately prepare for the academic rigor waiting for me in medical school.

In medical school, I studied constantly. I studied all day, every day, almost nonstop. Some might think us type A personality medical students are studying this hard to get ahead. But the reality is that we do it just to keep up with the volume of material thrown at us and often we still feel behind.

At the same time, we are human beings, not robots. We also must sleep, eat, and enjoy laughter in our lives. On the weekends, I did try to attend local events, work out, see friends, travel, and grab some extra sleep. It is difficult and humbling to work so hard while feeling I have not mastered anything, with more and more work routinely piled on.

I became more efficient at managing my time. I learned to take breaks to maintain my sanity. No matter how difficult things became, I was grateful to be a medical student. This path is not easy, but I chose it for a reason. I love learning about medicine and would not have it any other way. Medical school taught me that success is a series of small wins. You must decide what your highest priorities are and have the courage to say "no" to things that do not always serve your purpose. I learned that the road to medicine is a slow process, but quitting will not speed it up.

I face challenges. I feel my greatest challenge is having colleagues who lack the historical context of what centuries of structurally racist ideas and practices are present within the medical community that leads to African American distrust of the system. I cringe when I hear colleagues complain about a patient when they have no idea of the cultural differences. I, however, do not always find it my place to correct them. I hope my colleagues join me in meeting the needs of our patients and I can constructively help them understand their own implicit biases.

Another challenge is having my position questioned every day. It appears I should only be a housekeeper, or in dietary, or a nurse as a black female, even when I introduce myself as a doctor and part of the surgical team.

I find myself being questioned by patients, "Are you actually my doctor?" I also find myself being doubted by colleagues. I strive to prove them wrong. I am daily reminded of the need to intensify the call to action for augmented diversity in medicine. I do believe racism exists in medicine and many African American physicians have their individual stories about being ostracized because of the color of their skin. I may be known to some as a black female first and as a black female who has worked to achieve the privileges afforded a medical doctor secondly. I will continue to try to break down these barriers, one person at a time.

I feel resilience is like a muscle. Difficult times are never fun, but they are what make us stronger. The days as an intern will be long and difficult, but I want to remain authentic. I try to keep my human touch and do my best to ameliorate the pain, suffering, and misery of my patients, even if all I can do is offer a friendly conversation.

A typical day for me involves seeing patients and making sure I keep things in order for the rest of the team. I typically wake up around 4:30 a.m. and arrive at work by 5:30 a.m. I check my patients' charts and review labs, imaging results, notes, and more before seeing them. I round with the team and am updated on things we are doing for each patient throughout the day.

Depending on the service, I spend the middle part of my day assisting with floor work or assisting in the operating room. At the end of the day, I round again and make sure daily tasks have been completed. I arrive home around 6 p.m. and eat dinner, sometimes exercise, study, and am in bed around 10 p.m.

My greatest accomplishment/greatest or proudest moment was competing as the only junior in a world golf championship at Pebble Beach — twice! And the last non-medical book I read was *Girl, Wash Your Face,* by Rachel Hollis. My dream vacation is laying on a private beach in Bora Bora while sipping a tropical fruity drink!

The best advice I received was, "Decide what kind of life you really want, then say no to everything that isn't that."

The pearls of wisdom I would like to share with others are, "Never stop challenging yourself. The day you do, you are falling behind. You inspire people who pretend to not even see you, trust me. Right now you might be in a situation you think you will not survive, but six months ago you were in a situation you did not think you would survive and two years ago you were in a situation you did not think you would survive. The point is, you will always surprise yourself and you will ALWAYS make it through. Just keep swimming."

"I've missed more than 9000 shots in my career. I've lost almost 300 games. 26 times I've been trusted to take the game winning shot and missed. I've failed over and over and over again in my life. And that is why I succeed." – Michael Jordan

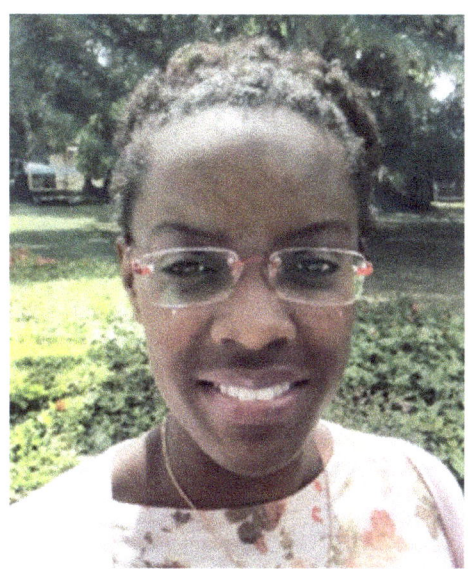

Dr. Rossana Chipalavela

Dr. Rossana Chipalavela is a pediatric surgery registrar (resident) at the Hospital Pioneiro Zeca, Lubango, Angola, Africa. She is currently completing her training in Kenya, Africa.

This is Dr. Chipalavela's story in her words.

When I was a child, I was always sick and spent a great deal of time in a pediatric hospital. I think the time I spent there created a deep passion inside of me to help others.

When I was in my third year in medical school, I went to the theater (operating room) for the first time to assist with a tracheostomy (creating a hole in the front of the throat of a patient) and this was the day I decided I wanted to become a surgeon. Since I love to work with children, I decided to pursue pediatric surgery.

On a typical day, I arrive at the hospital at 7 a.m. and time passes so quickly I realize patients are eating dinner and I have not had lunch yet! That is my typical day! We are busy taking care of patients in the unit and operating. The days go by ridiculously fast.

I find my greatest challenge is balancing personal life choices and career choices. This has been difficult. Also, I had to leave my country, Angola, and come to Kenya to pursue my dream. But the struggle is worth it when I see results.

I found an organization that works with cleft lip and palate defects and am able to work with them in my country. We perform free cleft surgery for both adults and children. When I watched a 52-year-old who spent her whole life with a bilateral cleft lip smile, it was one of the most amazing moments of my life. Currently, they are training me to do cleft surgery.

I build confidence by seeing examples of great brilliant women surgeons and what they have achieved. I always look at them and say to myself, "If they made it, I will also make it."

When failure or complications happen, I try to take the positive lessons I learn and apply them the next time I am in a similar situation.

I had a difficult time finding balance during my first year of residency and somehow this brought me closer to God. God is Who shows me how to balance.

Three people I would want to sit with and learn from are Jesus Christ. He is and will always be the greatest Doctor of all times. My mother. She is the most incredible woman I know. I don't know how she can do so much and never complains. She is my rock. And, Nelson Mandela. It is not easy to forgive people who hurt you, but it is even more difficult to still love someone who hurt you.

"You gain strength, courage and confidence by every experience in which you really stop to look fear in the face. You are able to say to yourself, 'I have lived through this horror. I can take the next thing that comes along.' You must do the thing you think you cannot do." – Eleanor Roosevelt

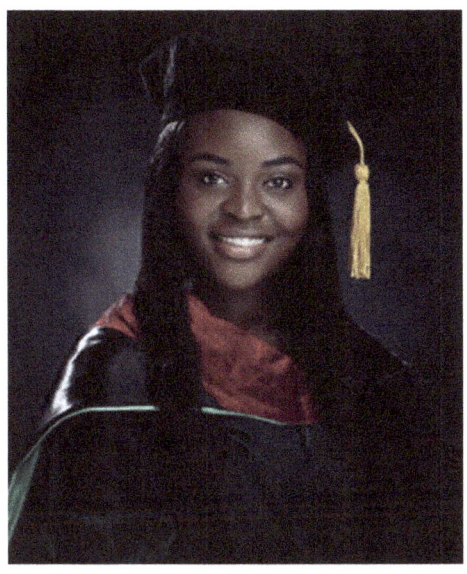

Dr. Sharon Cheryl Bonya

Dr. Sharon Cheryl Bonya is a surgical intern at Kamuzu Central Hospital, Lilongwe, Central Region, Malawi, Africa. She earned her bachelor's degree from Southwestern University in Cebu, Philippines and her medical degree from Emilio Aguinaldo College in Manila, Philippines.

This is Dr. Bonya's story in her words. Perils of studying abroad.

"Where did you study?" she asked, giggling. One of the consults asked me this at the Kamuzu Central Hospital where I am completing my post-graduate internship. My colleague and I were doing morning ward rounds along with other doctors. Both of us studied medicine outside of Malawi.

We answered her with enthusiasm clearly stating where we studied. Her reply was rude and insulting. My colleague and I looked at each other, blankly, unsure of what she meant or why she was treating me this way. We had only been in the department for a few weeks when we met this consultant. Her insolent stereotypical statements did not infuriate me because I had endured such remarks from others.

At age 10, I moved from Malawi to the United States of America. Since I went to middle school and high school in America, I knew what diversity, prejudice, and racism meant. Being an African and a girl in such an environment was not easy, but I made it through.

I will fast forward to my years in medical school. I was a Malawian-born, American-raised woman, embarking on a journey in a new country in Asia, the Philippines, to pursue my medical degree. Things were not smooth here either.

The language barrier was one thing; colossal racism was another. I endured all of it. Often, I called my parents, who were thousands of miles away, to tell them I wanted to quit. All they could do is encourage me as any parent would.

In my final year of medical school, I rotated through the different medical and surgical services at the hospital daily and experienced patient care firsthand. Learning from my senior interns as well as residents and consultants was a great experience. But I felt lost because I was one of the five Africans in my class and the only Malawian.

Despite the discrimination I experienced from several colleagues as well as patients and their families, I did not give up. I still received a proper medical education that I will be able to use for the rest of my life. I would not trade this experience for anything because I learned to fix my eyes on my ultimate goal despite the challenges and obstacles I faced. I was even more motivated by the love and support I received from the senior interns, residents, and consultants who did believe in me.

I have not only become more proficient in my practical skills, but, because of my experiences, I have also become better at dealing with people as an intern medical officer at the Central Hospital in the capital city of Malawi.

Another encounter I had was with the consultant at Kamuzu Central Hospital. I do not know if it is the way I look or the way I speak, no one knows but her, but she also was rude to me. Sometimes others feel that since I am Malawian I lack medical knowledge and am, therefore, incompetent to diagnose and treat patients. Thus, I am labeled as such. I often find myself overworking to prove that I am as good as they are or, at times, even better.

In the end, however, it all depends on the environment in which you surround yourself. I choose positivity every day. I start my day with God to help me through challenges and obstacles each day, as well as end my day with Him. Always remember, you can build a solid foundation with the same bricks others use to throw at you.

What I would tell myself in grade school is, "Enjoy life. Make friends." What I would tell myself in middle school is, "Growing up is a trap, do not get too excited. Just kidding!" What I would tell myself in high school is, "Become the best version of yourself. Have fun, however, remember that your academic life is important." What I would tell myself in undergrad is, "Be present and avoid distractions. Life only gets tougher." What I would tell myself in medical school is, "You probably want to give up. Learning human anatomy and pathology is not easy, but you can and will do it." What I would tell myself before starting my internship is, "Ignore the mean seniors and patients. Learn and make mistakes while you are still under supervision."

"When I stand before God at the end of my life, I would hope that I would not have a single bit of talent left, and could say, 'I used everything you gave me.'" – Erma Bombeck

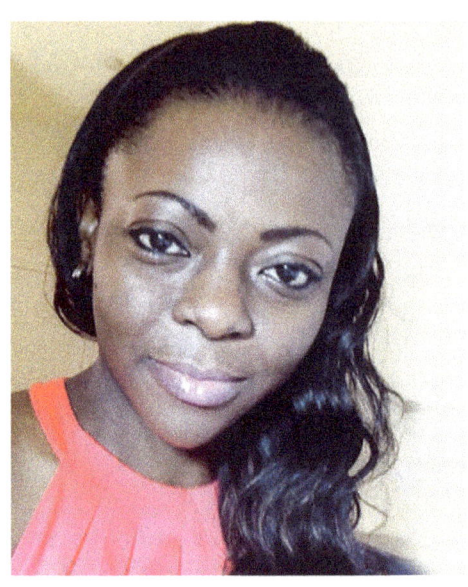

Dr. Nadege Fackche

Dr. Nadege Fackche is a general surgery resident at Howard University Hospital in Washington, D.C. She completed her undergraduate degree in respiratory therapy at the University of South Dakota, Vermillion, and earned her medical degree at the University of South Carolina, School of Medicine, Columbia. She completed a two-year surgical oncology post-doctoral research fellowship at John Hopkins University in Baltimore, Maryland.

This is Dr. Fackche's story.

My father is a professor of math and was very intentional in letting me and my sisters know that it was important for us to be well-educated and self-sufficient and not rely on a man to provide for us. I have three sisters that are well-to-do and educated.

My grandmother was a non-compliant diabetic, meaning she did not follow doctors' directions to manage her high blood sugars. I accompanied her to doctors' appointments when I was a child and this exposure to the medical field influenced my decision to become a doctor when I was six years old.

When I was a young girl, I asked my father what the highest degree was that one can attain. He told me a doctorate was the highest degree. So, I knew from that young age I had to earn a doctorate. I started my medical school training in my home country, Cameroon, Africa, and one of my uncles who is an ophthalmologist in Virginia, wanted me to come and study in the United States. So, he and my parents made the decision for me to study in the States. I was not involved in the decision making. They made the arrangements for me to attend the University of South Dakota.

I moved to the States in January and it was a huge adjustment. I found myself trying to figure things out as I completed my undergraduate training. It was different from how medical training is structured in Cameroon. My parents were not wealthy, so they could not pay for my tuition. My parents did not realize how expensive it is to attend school in the States. To this day, my father tells me that if he knew how difficult it would be financially and how expensive schooling is, he would not have made the arrangements for me to come to the States. I am glad he made the choices he did because everything worked out well.

I earned my undergraduate degree in respiratory therapy because this allowed me to work to support myself while pursuing my medical degree. I had a boyfriend when I was in Cameroon, but I did not think it was a serious relationship because I never saw myself as the marrying type or the kind of woman to have children. I imagined I would focus on my career as a doctor.

But God had other plans because our relationship became serious after I moved to South Dakota. We married and arranged for him to move to the States permanently. I worked for five years as a respiratory therapist and enjoyed my work while I prepared to apply to medical school and financial aid.

I considered a career in pulmonary critical care after completing medical school, but during my general surgery rotation, I fell in love with surgery. By the time I started medical school, I had two young children and wondered if I would be able to be a surgeon, a wife, and a mother. I realized after rotating through all the services in medicine, including OB/GYN and the emergency room, nothing made me as happy as surgery. My husband was instrumental in my decision to choose surgery because he noticed how much I loved being in surgery and how I felt about my other rotations. He promised he would be supportive and help me achieve my goal of becoming a surgeon.

I did my sub-internship (sub-I) in head and neck cancer surgery at Brigham and Women's Hospital in Boston, Massachusetts, when I was seven months pregnant with our third baby. It was an amazing experience and I was nicely supported during this rotation. I worked hard and enjoyed every moment of my sub-I. I was at the forefront of cutting-edge surgical procedures and pushing the boundaries of science, medicine, and surgery. It was amazing for me.

We spent a great deal of time in the operating room doing ground-breaking surgery and I was in awe. While I was there, I realized I wanted to pursue surgical oncology. It is an exciting field and there is still much to learn in this area. My purpose is to improve cancer care for patients.

What drives me at this time is that there is an entire race of people, black people, which has not been studied in terms of cancer treatment and research. Different cancers affect black people differently from other races, and I want to contribute to how we can optimize treatment for this group of people.

To recap my education in a nutshell, I completed my undergraduate schooling at the University of South Dakota and my medical school training at the University of South Carolina, School of Medicine. I matched at Howard University Hospital, Washington, D.C., for my general surgery residency. I recently completed a two-year research fellowship at Johns Hopkins University in Baltimore, Maryland, between my second and third clinical years. I returned to Howard and am in my third year of clinical residency training.

When I was applying for residency, I was intentional about where I wanted to train. Howard University was my first choice because when I met Dr. Lori Wilson, the program director for the general surgery residency there, I knew she would support me and be a great mentor. She is a mother and wife as well as an excellent surgeon. It was important to have a great support system of other mothers who understand what you are going through because I suffered a great deal with mom guilt. My children are 12, 10, 7, and 5 years old. It has been a challenge to raise children while training to be a surgeon. This is where your village comes in, having a supportive partner and others to assist as needed and help with childcare when necessary.

As far as balance goes, I think there is no balance. There are times I need to focus on my school work and there are times I set my school work aside so I can focus on my family. There will never be balance for me, and that's alright with me. My greatest concern is to make certain to check in with my family frequently, especially my husband. Communication is important.

I love to cook and I often bake with my children, which is a great time to bond. During this season of life, my husband does most of the child-rearing. I make sure there are meals cooked days in advance to help lighten his load. We work well together to keep our home functioning well and thriving. I gave up the idea that I am in control of everything and this has helped to decrease the stress.

The best advice I received is, "You must own your story. Stop trying to make your story fit into other people's boxes. Be who you are and the people who matter will value you for being yourself. Do not try to be someone you are not so you can fit in or so you can be liked."

How I find strength is I pray a great deal of the time. When things are difficult, I give myself permission to cry. Then, I pray and move on. Having the complete support of my husband and children gives me strength each day. They are my reason for doing all that I do.

The lessons I would like to share with those coming up the ranks are, "Dream big. There will be obstacles, but you must fight hard to have the life you want. A support system is crucial to your success. You cannot live on an island. You need people who will encourage you along the journey. Networking is important. I used to believe hard work was enough to help you advance, but hard work alone is not enough. You need people who will open doors of opportunity for you."

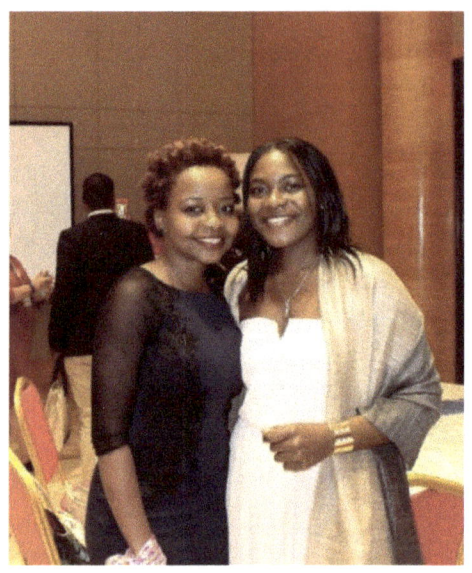

Dr. Busi Mlambo (left) Dr. Pamela Samoyo (right)

Dr. Busi Mlambo is a registrar (resident) in general surgery at the University of Zimbabwe in Zimbabwe, Africa. She earned a bachelor's degree in molecular biology, bioinformatics, and biochemistry at the University of Maryland, College Park in the USA, and a bachelor of medicine and surgery from the University of Witwatersrand in Johannesburg, South Africa. She is a proud member of Women in Surgery Africa (WISA) and passionate about playing her part in empowering women in surgery.

Dr. Mlambo was born and raised in Bulawayo, Zimbabwe. She attended junior high and high school there. Her mom was a midwife when Dr. Mlambo was born, but her mother furthered her education in the medical field to attain additional qualifications in public health and adult education.

Her stepfather was a general practitioner. Dr. Mlambo feels our career paths are often guided by our areas of academic strength. However, when she reached her O-level training, she discovered she loved and excelled in both arts and crafts and sciences. As a result, the school referred her to a psychologist for career guidance counseling. The psychologist analyzed Dr. Mlambo and concluded she was suited for the medical field, particularly an area of medicine in which Dr. Mlambo would be able to use her hands.

The two recommendations highlighted were surgery and dentistry. Dr. Mlambo believes the combination of being raised by parents in the medical field and the results of this psychological evaluation set in place the first cobblestones on the path that led her to where she is today.

Dr. Mlambo chose surgery because she thinks surgery is the perfect balance between science and art. This is clearly where she belongs, somewhere in the middle of the two. Time flies when she is in the theater (operating room). Dr. Mlambo loses all sense of herself and is focused only on the task before her. She has a calm and rejuvenating feeling when she leaves the external pressures and stresses outside the theater and surrenders her mind and hands to the patient on the operating table.

Another reason she chose general surgery was her fear of regret. Dr. Mlambo worried she would regret not having followed her dreams had she chosen a different profession. One may ask, "Why should she have felt pressured to choose a different profession?" Because she knew surgery would not be a walk in the park for a married woman with children. She knew the demands of this career path and how the time commitment diverts time from family. Dr. Mlambo worried about the potential ramifications. She tried to investigate other less taxing careers.

She considered radiology, which has been dubbed an ideal specialty for women because it provides a rewarding lifestyle and the option of working from home. However, she found it unbearable to think she would not interact with patients.

Dr. Mlambo believes the close relationship between a surgeon and his or her patient begins the moment an initial history is taken and the patient is examined. She believes this relationship continues through ward rounds and clinic visits for follow-up care and is vital for the patient's well-being and holistic management of the patient. Dr. Mlambo feels this is vital for the surgeon as well. Her life would feel incomplete if her interaction with a patient began and ended in the theater or with the interpretation of their radiological imaging. She needs to know the person behind the images. She wants to know why they presented, why she made certain decisions about their treatment, how they progressed, and what their outcome was. Dr. Mlambo wants to know how she can build on the knowledge she gained to help other patients going forward.

When she accepted all these things about herself, she knew her career had to be surgery. Dr. Mlambo explored traditionally female-friendly disciplines like ENT (ear/nose/throat), which she rotated through for six months hoping to fall in love with the specialty, but general surgery maintained its fierce grip on her heart.

Although she experienced some racism in her medical training in South Africa, Dr. Mlambo cannot say it scarred her for life. She quickly learned as a black female that if she stayed on top of her game, spoke out, and answered questions correctly and confidently, the color of her skin faded into the background. When the bedside tutorial seemed directed more towards her fairer-skinned colleagues, she engaged the lecturers with challenging questions or answered questioned in a manner impressive enough to re-focus the conversation. This resulted in her receiving the full benefit of the tutorial and future tutorials as well. Dr. Mlambo quickly learned that when the odds are not stacked in your favor, you have to stick your neck out much further to achieve an A in life, so this is exactly what she did and she succeeded.

Dr. Mlambo married a supportive husband who has

backed her career choices since her final year in medical school. She had their firstborn son during her second year of internship, one and a half years before beginning surgical training. Internship in Zimbabwe varies from two to four years.

She had their second baby, a girl, during her third year of surgical training. Being a registrar (resident) in surgical training with two young children has been difficult because of the long hours she spends at the hospital. There is mom guilt associated with many working mothers, wondering if they spend enough time with their children?

Dr. Mlambo thinks comparison is the thief of joy. She tries not to dwell on this but at times she cannot help comparing herself to male colleagues because they have more time to read since their wives are at home caring for their children and homemaking. It is unrealistic to compare yourself to people who are different from you. For instance, one night she spent two hours trying to help the baby to sleep because she was fussy. Some nights her children needed to be breastfed several times during the night.

Also, there have been times one of her children was sick and she was up most of the night caring for them. Though she has support, when her children are sick, they want their mom. Finding balance has been challenging and she cannot say for sure she ever will find balance.

When she has difficult days in training, Dr. Mlambo finds the strength to keep going from colleagues at work. She feels everyone should know their team and not be afraid to call for help. She has mentors and keeps their numbers on speed dial. She needs someone to ask, "Did I do the right thing here? What would you have done? Should I have done anything differently?" She learns from experiences.

Dr. Mlambo keeps her family informed of when she will be home. She talks to her husband or her mom about challenging situations. And she remembers that through everything, it is important to maintain patient confidentiality and never provide information that could lead to the recognition or singling out of any patient.

She feels confidence relates to personality factors, and Dr. Mlambo is a type-A personality and an extrovert. So, confidence is not something she struggles with. As a matter of fact, confident is a word many people use to describe her, whether it is how she carries herself or how she answers questions. It is not something she focuses on or consciously puts on. She does think there are things anyone can do to make themselves feel more confident. These things are different for each person.

Dr. Mlambo feels dressing a certain way and presenting herself a certain way gives her confidence. So, on days she is not wearing scrubs, she dresses formally for her ward rounds and feels this boosts her confidence. Most importantly, she stays on top of her game. This means she knows her theory and she is operating well in the theater. This instills self-confidence, not only in herself but also in the consultants around her. This is vital in surgical training which is so mentorship-based.

If Dr. Mlambo had to choose one surgery to do and only one, she would have to say she would do a surgical oncology procedure because she makes meaningful and measurable differences in someone's life every day of her life. If she had to narrow it down even further, she would say surgical breast oncology, particularly the breast-conserving procedures where she rids women of their cancers while giving them the option of saving their breast. This translates into a preserved body image and beauty to many women.

She loves to play music in surgery. Yes, yes, and yes. She listens to anything and everything. Her theater playlist has a wide range of music ranging from artists such as Bob Marley to Maroon 5.

Dr. Mlambo will be the first to admit she has not done well finding balance. Most of the time, work comes first and everything else falls into place in whatever time is left over. Perhaps she should award herself with some protected time, be it an hour or two each day or a day of the week; time she commits to the people and activities that matter most to her outside work. It sounds close to impossible, especially for a surgeon in training; but it is possible. Dr. Mlambo loves to read but this is a difficult time to read for leisure because she has exams soon. The next book on her list is *This is Going to Hurt: The Secret Diaries of a Junior Doctor* by Adam Kay.

Lessons Dr. Mlambo shared are, "Manage time well. Everyone in the world has the same 24 hours a day you do. Apparently, there is a way to have it all as you maintain a balance between family and work, looking after yourself, exercising, and eating healthy food. When you figure this out, be sure to let me in on your secret! Keep your friends close and your family closer. You will need a social support system to get through surgical training. Get lots and lots and lots of help!! This may be in the form of help with childcare. Sometimes grandma's and grandpa's help with children. Keep your key people in the loop and informed about upcoming hurdles or challenges so they can anticipate any added stress you may be experiencing. For example, I told my husband ahead of time when my next rotation would be difficult. I informed him when I would be on call every weekend for six months and would be unable to do anything on weekends, including traveling. I informed him when I would only be home in the evenings. This helped him prepare for the difficult months, so he did not feel blind-sided and was able to deal with my absences and remain supportive. Ultimately, and most importantly, just do the best you can. Friends and family know they do not see me at family functions, and this is ok. Sometimes I miss my children's school events, and this is ok. I am not perfect, but I do the best I can! And finally, if you worry that a part of you will always be incomplete if you do not become a surgeon, then you must do this. The decision you must make here and now is to become a surgeon. As for the how, figure it out as you go. That is it!"

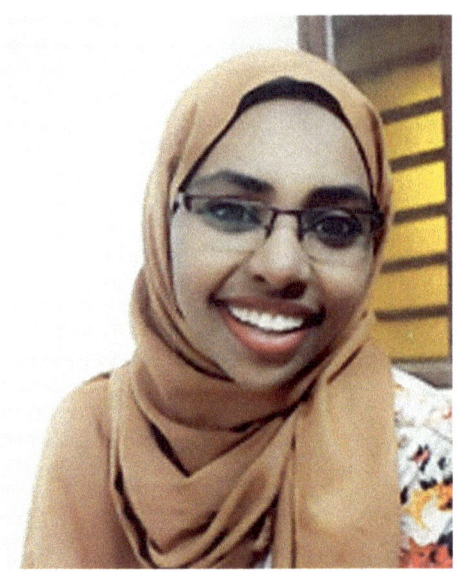

Dr. Eman Abdel Azim Elsadek Elhassan

Dr. Eman Abdel Azim Elsadek Elhassan is a fifth-year surgical resident from Sudan. She is a member of the Royal College of Surgeons, Edinburgh (MRCS-Ed). She received her medical degree from the Upper Nile University in South Sudan, Africa.

This is Dr. Adbel Azim Elsadek Elhassan's story in her words.

I chose a career in medicine because my father is a doctor. I loved seeing him in a white coat with a stethoscope around his neck. During my medical school surgical rotation, I fell in love with surgery because of the fine motor skills necessary for surgery and the gentleness of surgery. Since it seems surgery is a male-dominated field and some women in my country of Sudan, for cultural and religious reasons, prefer a female surgeon, I feel I can offer them my expertise.

The challenges I face are working in a field with male predominance. Also, like other developing countries, we have a brain-drain where our highly trained professionals leave the country, and we are left without adequate staff. And, something that may be different for us is we do not have adequate call-rooms and healthy food making it challenging when working more than 24-hour shifts.

My greatest accomplishment and my greatest or proudest moments are when I see the junior doctors I teach excelling and doing well. This makes me enormously proud. Also, I was proud when I was admitted as a full member of the Royal College of Surgeons [MRCS] and received my certificate at the ceremony. I was so happy because I saw the pride on my parents' faces. My greatest achievement will be when I pass my final exam in a few months and officially become a surgeon.

The best advice I have received is "Read, read, and read as much as you can."

As far a finding balance goes, I am deeply convinced that God has a plan for my life, and He is in control of everything that happens. I remember when I was pregnant, I struggled due to the physiological changes of pregnancy. I waited for hours for public transportation to reach the hospital on time for my shift. I struggled with shortness of breath and fatigue. While standing for an hour or two doing a thyroidectomy or any other operation I experienced swelling in my legs. I remember the thirst I felt that drove me to drink three liters of water in one sitting. And then, my daughter decided it was time to be born when I was preparing to operate. Everything worked out well.

After she was born, I worked day and night, including weekends and holidays, to offer the best for my family. Now, I am studying for my final exam, holding my thesis in one hand and carrying my daughter with the other. It is not easy to find balance and I have accepted this. I am determined to be successful in all areas of my life. In my spare time I play the piano and write books.

Three people I would like to have dinner with and learn from are Benjamin Carson (American neurosurgeon), Maria Siemionow (Polish transplant female surgeon), and Reem Balilah (Sudanese hepatobiliary female surgeon).

Lessons I would like to share with the up-and-coming young black female surgeon are, "Being a surgeon is an amazing career. Do not shy away from it if it is what you desire to do. There will be people who do not support you along your journey to becoming a surgeon, but do not allow this to stop you. Let your personal life be parallel to your surgical career. There is no better time to get married, be a mother, and continue productive relationships with your friends and family. You will struggle much in your surgical career, but whenever you fall, you must find a way to get back up on your feet and keep going."

"You walk one step at a time, and so you must achieve milestones one at a time, whatever your role in life turns out to be."
– Kathryn Anderson, MD

CHAPTER TWENTY-THREE
My Story

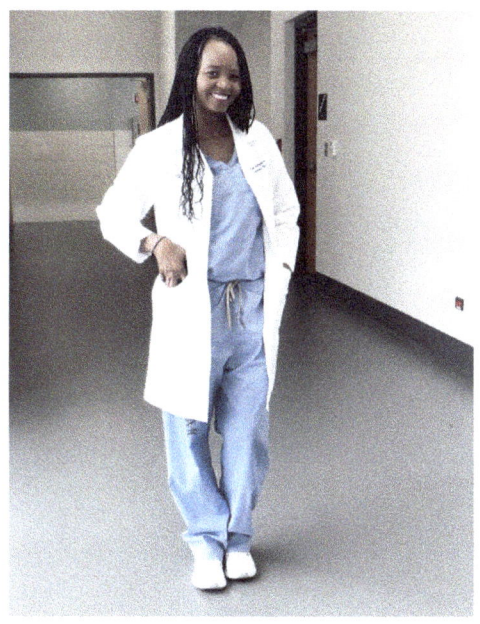

Dr. Praise Matemavi

For as long as I can remember, I wanted to be a doctor. When I was six years old, a medical team from Loma Linda University Medical Center, Loma Linda, California, came to my home country, Zimbabwe, to help start the open-heart surgery program at Parirenyatwa Hospital.

My father told me about this project and from this time on, my goal was to become a heart surgeon. We often drove by the hospital and I looked at the intimidating buildings that made-up one of the world's largest hospitals at that time, with more than 5000 beds. I imagined myself grown up, dressed in my white coat, and taking care of patients.

My parents encouraged my dream and in fifth grade one of my birthday gifts was the book *Gifted Hands* by Dr. Ben

Carson. I devoured the pages in one sitting. I was enthralled by the mysteries of medicine and surgery.

We moved to the United States of America when I was 14 years old. It was a cold and snowy day in mid-December when we landed at the O'Hare International Airport, Chicago, Illinois. I have always disliked cold and I never saw snow before but adapted quickly to our new home in Michigan on the campus of Andrews University where my father was studying for his master's in divinity.

Being a pastor's child, we moved many times. By the time we moved to Michigan, I had already attended six different schools, so it was an easy adjustment. Berrien Springs is a small village, population 1800. It is best known for being a Seventh - Day Adventist community. Muhammad Ali lived in our quiet, safe village that had two traffic lights and no Walmart. I loved the intimacy of my new community compared to the hustle and bustle of living in the outskirts of Harare, the capital city of Zimbabwe. I quickly made friends with other girls who lived on campus whose parents were also studying at Andrews University.

High school was fun and a breeze for me. I found the American education system much easier than the British education system I came from. American education was structured with study guides and multiple-choice questions and the British education system consisted of essay and problem-solving testing.

We did not have money for me to attend the university, but I had dreams and intelligence on my side. I enrolled in a community college where I was blessed with scholarships to cover my tuition. I planned to complete my prerequisites for a biology degree while working full-time to save money for university costs. As an international student, I was not eligible for student loans and the resources available to me were limited.

At age 18, I became pregnant. It was a devastating blow to me and my parents, who migrated to the United States so I could have the opportunities and resources necessary to follow my dreams of becoming a heart surgeon. This was the beginning of a difficult four-year period in my life.

I became a victim of domestic violence and later, a survivor. I felt alone despite having close family and friends who cared about me. I hid my pain. I was ashamed. During this time, I changed my course of study and completed my associate degree in nursing and was blessed with a second child.

By age 23, I was working full-time as a cardiac telemetry nurse and raising two beautiful children as a single mother. I was blessed to have the unwavering support of my parents and sister, however, my dream of medicine never died. Every time I encountered female physicians, it fueled my drive.

With sheer determination and hard work, I completed my prerequisites for medical school in two semesters. I took general chemistry, organic chemistry, biology, and physics at the same time I studied for the medical college admission test (MCAT).

By God's grace, I did well on the MCAT and applied to medical schools. I did not have an adviser. I researched and figured everything myself. I knew I needed a bachelor's degree to be accepted to medical school, so I enrolled in the university affiliated with our community college. I was able to complete the required 60 credits in one year! I was accepted to every medical school I applied to and chose my home-state medical school.

When I was 14 years old, shortly after arriving in the states, a family friend drove me and my sister to Michigan State University. It was a sunny Saturday afternoon and we saw the beautiful campus and toured East Lansing.

I am uncertain if our friend was considering attending Michigan State University or what her motivation was for taking the trip. We walked around the campus and when we arrived at the administration building with the big green S, my sister took a photo of me standing on the S. I wrote on the back of the photo, "This is where I will come for medical school someday." This was one of many instances in my life I had a vision of exactly what I wanted and years later, it happened.

When the time came to apply for residency training, I applied to both allopathic and osteopathic surgical residencies. At the time I was applying for residency, the osteopathic and allopathic matches were at different times. The osteopathic match (DO) was in February and the allopathic match (MD) was in March. For osteopathic medical students applying to both osteopathic and allopathic residency programs, we had the opportunity to take advantage of the allopathic match if we did not match into a residency in the osteopathic match. Though I interviewed for 12 osteopathic surgical residencies, I only wanted to train at Sinai Grace Hospital in Detroit, Michigan, and if I did not match there, then I would participate in the allopathic match. It was my heart's desire to train at Sinai Grace Hospital, Detroit Medical Center, Detroit, Michigan, and I matched at Sinai Grace and completed my internship year.

Three days after graduating from medical school, I married a wonderful man I met in medical school. He, however, matched in neurosurgery in New York. It was a difficult year for our marriage because we were both in demanding residencies. The following year I relocated to New York for general surgery training at New York Presbyterian Queens Hospital in Flushing, New York. This was one of the best decisions I made.

My surgical residency was difficult and during my third year of training, we divorced. It was another dark and difficult period in my life. I slowly drifted from God, though I continued to say my prayers. My relationship with God was at its lowest point. It was during this dark time I rebuilt my relationship with my Creator. I needed His strength to get out of bed and make it through the difficult days.

I put a smile on my face and continued to work hard, learning how to be the best surgeon I could be. I had a 10-minute walk to work and used this time to talk to God and listen to uplifting Christian music. Eventually, I began to heal and rebuild my life as a single mother again. God has shown me time and again that His grace is sufficient for me. I forged through the fourth year of surgical residency without many incidences. This is a year you have the opportunity to operate a great deal and it was amazing.

In the second half of my fourth year I applied for a transplant surgery fellowship. I traveled the country, interviewing at phenomenal programs. Through all the travels and interviews, my heart set on a fellowship at the University of Nebraska Medical Center in Omaha, Nebraska. This was my last interview.

When I was a second-year medical student at Michigan State University, a professor once saw me reading a book about a pediatric cardio-thoracic surgeon called, *Walk on Water: The Miracle of Saving Children's Lives* by Michael Ruhlman. This professor said that to him, the only other surgery that was technically challenging and beautiful in its own right, was a pediatric liver transplant surgery. He knew a surgeon who did this named Dr. Alan Langnas in Nebraska.

That day, I researched all I could about liver transplants and decided that I would work hard so that I could go to Nebraska to train to become a transplant surgeon under Dr. Langnas' tutelage. You can imagine how excited I was to open my email that June afternoon eight years later as I sat in Central Park to find out that I was matched with Nebraska for my fellowship training. This was by far one of the best days of my life!

I breezed through the first half of my chief resident year, my last year of residency, but three months before my graduation, I faced another dark period. My beautiful mother, who was my prayer warrior and the president of my fan club, was diagnosed with extremely aggressive triple-negative breast cancer. She died within one month of her diagnosis.

I was devastated and had many regrets because I did not realize her time on this earth was this short. I regretted not spending time with her at the end of her life. I took one week off after her funeral and returned to work, business as usual. I dug deep within myself to find the strength to continue each day even though all I wanted to do was cry.

Each time I saw a patient on a ventilator, it brought back memories of her last few hours before we disconnected the ventilator and made sure she was comfortable. During this painful time, I developed a deep respect and appreciation for palliative care physicians. God saw me through, and I graduated from residency and relocated to Nebraska for the ride of a lifetime.

Fellowship was a beast. Nothing prepared me for the long surgeries and even longer days. Also, the flights in private jets to various hospitals around the country, often arriving in the middle of the night, leaving with precious lifesaving and life-altering organs for our patients, was something new to me.

I worked with the most amazing team and grew professionally and personally more than I ever thought possible. Even with the long hours and busyness, I managed to meet the love of my life. He has been a great support and friend. Often, I look back at my journey and marvel at how God led me each step of the way. Even in my darkest days, He was there.

It has been an amazing journey and I see the hand of God in every step, especially during my darkest moments. I have had the opportunity to meet many amazing people along the way, men and women who believed in me and opened doors for me.

In this season in my life, I am exactly where I am supposed to be. I feel extremely blessed to have incredible partners in my practice who support me and have made my transition as an attending smooth. I am grateful for all the trials and tribulations, for they too have shaped the woman I am today. I would not be where I am today was it not for my family and friends who have been through thick-and-thin with me, always encouraging me to keep going. It truly took a village to produce the first Zimbabwean multi-visceral transplant surgeon.

A note about some of the women in this book.

Along the way, I found friend after friend. Now, I am sincerely grateful to each and every one of them for helping me tell my story and theirs.

It was a pleasure and amazing opportunity to talk with Mr. and Mrs. Gordon about their daughter, Dr. Sherilyn Gordon-Burroughs. Dr. Sherilyn died three months before I graduated from my surgical residency and began my multi-organ transplant surgery fellowship. I never met her, but I knew about her because there were only six black female transplant surgeons practicing in the United States at that time. She was the third trained in abdominal transplant surgery. Being such a small group of black female surgeons, everyone knows one another. As I write this book, there are 10 practicing black female transplant surgeons. I hope there will be many more in the years to come! I believe anyone with a dream can have it come true. I want Dr. Sherilyn Gordon-Burroughs to be remembered for the amazing and strong woman she was and thank her for her inspiration.

Dr. Sherilyn Gordon-Burroughs and I share our experiences with domestic violence. I want to share her story in this collection to ensure she is not forgotten. I am also a victim of domestic violence and in my journey to healing, I met some incredible women who share this with us.

Another beautiful woman I have had the pleasure of meeting is Dr. Arika Hoffman. I first met her when I interviewed for my transplant surgery fellowship at the University of Nebraska Medical Center in Omaha. We had many things in common and quickly became close friends. We are both from Michigan and discovered we knew many of the same people. This made talking easy and we naturally found something to talk about all the time.

Also, both our mothers died the same year and we understood each other's grief. When I needed to go home to California in an emergency, she quickly booked a plane ticket for me to leave that day. She has been a mentor, sponsor, confidant, and, most of all, a friend.

And another of my favorite women is Dr. Velma Scantlebury. The first time I met Dr. Scantlebury was at the society of black academic surgeons meeting in Birmingham, Alabama, in 2018. I knew she would be attending and was looking forward to meeting her. I had been corresponding with her for four years via email prior to our meeting.

When I was a third-year general surgery resident, I emailed her telling her I wanted to be a transplant surgeon and asked for advice. She emailed back that same day and from then on mentored me through residency and fellowship and now as a new attending. She is always so well-dressed and put together. I love shoes and can always tell a fellow shoe-lover. I can only imagine what her shoe closet looks like! She is the first black female transplant surgeon in the United States of America. She is a wonderful mentor and my hero!

I researched everything about Dr. Scantlebury when I was a medical student, watched every interview, and read every interview. I also read her autobiography in one day when I was on vacation. I feel I know her life story. I know she wanted to be a doctor since she was seven years old and moved to the United States when she was 15 years old from Barbados. I always wondered what this was like.

Dr. Scantlebury was trained by Dr. Starzl, who is considered the father of liver transplant surgery. I read his memoir, *The Puzzle People* multiple times. I was sad when he retired before I was ready to train in transplant surgery. Because I trained at the University of Nebraska Medical Center, I feel I have a little piece of him since he trained Dr. Bud Shaw who trained Dr. Alan Langnas, who trained me. I consider Dr. Langnas my father of transplant surgery.

Another phenomenal surgeon I admire is Dr. Patricia Turner. I first met her when I was a second-year surgical resident. One of my mentors, Dr. Armando Castro, introduced us at an American College of Surgeons Leadership and Advocacy Summit. There were no surgeons who looked like me in my home institution and he made it a point to connect me with her. She does not know this, but throughout my training, she was a surgical idol of mine.

I followed her rising career with enthusiasm and excitement to see a beautiful black woman surgeon accomplishing so much, giving me hope for what I could accomplish in my career.

I remember leaning in and listening to her intently each time she spoke, whether it was in a large conference room or at the networking dinners. She is the epitome of black girl magic. I love how humble she is and how hard she works to make sure that underrepresented minorities' voices are heard. I could sit and talk with her all day and bask in her wisdom. I was pleased when I told her I was writing a book as a tribute to Dr. Sherilyn Gordon Burroughs and she was happy to be a contributor.

Dr. Iyore James is also dear to me. When I prepared for my general surgery oral boards, I told her how nervous I was to take this difficult exam since I had been in transplant surgery training for two years and not done general surgery and trauma surgery for that long, which was what would be asked. She took time out of her schedule to coach me and review cases two days before the exam. She is a great friend and mentor.

My first time at the Society of Black Academic Surgeons Scientific Session in 2018 which was held at University of Alabama in Birmingham, Alabama, I had never seen so many black female surgeons in one room before. I thought to myself, "Wow, these amazing, beautiful black women are excelling in this male-dominated field." I stood at the edge of the room with my mentor and friend, Dr. Arika Hoffman, because I wanted to take it all in. I trained at an institution where I was the only black categorical surgical resident in the six years I was there and there was only one male African American surgeon who was in private practice. So, one can imagine how excited I was to be in the same room with women in my field who looked like me.

As I stood there in awe of my colleagues, Dr. Zaria Murrell walked into the room. She had an energy about her I admired. I leaned over to my friend and said, "I have to know who that woman is."

I watched this woman who was the epitome of grace, style, elegance, and unmistakably a powerhouse. I learned she was a pediatric surgeon and I was slightly intimidated. Pediatric surgery is one of the most competitive surgical fellowships one can be accepted into and to me, they are the true general surgeons because they cover such a wide breadth of surgical disease processes. Their range is anything from thoracic (lung) surgeries to abdominal surgeries to the skin and soft tissue surgeries. I worked up the courage to approach her and ask to interview her for my book. She was warm and gracious to me. I enjoyed chatting with her and by the end of the interview, I was blown away by her tenacity, authenticity, and just how extraordinary she was.

Dr. Miriam Mutebi is a great friend and supporter. When I told her I was writing this book and including stories and interviews of black female surgeons, she was the first one on board with the project. She helped me contact the women in the Pan African Women Association of Surgeons. She is a powerhouse: the epitome of a triple achiever; a surgeon, a scientist, and an educator. She also has an amazing fashion sense and we share a love for beautiful shoes.

I was introduced to Dr. Portia Siwawa by a friend of mine Dr. Tobe Momah. Dr. Momah is a physician at the same hospital where I work. He was the first to welcome me to Jackson, Mississippi, and he and his wife have been a great resource for me and my family. When I mentioned I was creating a book about black female surgeons, he told me a friend he met during his residency was a surgeon from Botswana and helped me contact her. It was great to talk to my neighbor (Zimbabwe and Botswana are neighbors) who was an African girl-child who also survived surgical training in the Big Apple!

Dr. Violet Onkoba is one of my best friends. It is funny how we met. I was a fourth-year medical student applying for my general surgery residency. I wanted to train at Sinai Grace in Detroit, so I decided to make an appointment with Dr. William Anderson, a nationally known general surgeon and civil rights leader who, at the time, was the Vice President of Academic Affairs in Osteopathic Medical Education at Sinai Grace Hospital. I was given an hour of his time and went intending to consider the different osteopathic general surgery residencies and deciding which ones I would interview for. I had been granted interviews at more than 20 osteopathic surgical residencies and needed to narrow my list to 12.

After talking for a short time, he paged Dr. Onkoba to come to his office so I could meet her because he said to me, "You cannot be what you cannot see." I never met a black female general surgeon or resident, so what he did for me was not only tell me that it is possible, but he also showed me it is possible. I matched at Sinai Grace for general surgery training. We discovered we had much in common and became close over time. She is one-of-a-kind and I am grateful to call her my sister and my friend!

I cannot remember how I discovered Dr. Omofolasade Kosoko-Lasaki on the internet during my first year as a fellow in Nebraska, but I am glad I did. I emailed her asking to meet with her at her office. She responded graciously. She was not working in the same institution I was, so I drove downtown to her office at the Creighton University in Omaha, Nebraska, where she is the associate vice provost of the Health Sciences Multicultural and Community Affairs (HS-MACA) Department.

As we talked, I wanted to absorb everything she said. She taught me many lessons in the hour I spent with her. I could go on and on listing her accomplishments. She is an amazing woman and I am proud to call her my mentor. When I was an avid blogger, she is the one who inspired me to turn my blog posts into a book someday. Well, this is that book!

And I do not want to miss the opportunity to thank Dr. Lori Wilson. As I watched her documentary, I cried because I lost my mother to triple negative breast cancer. Her story hit very close to home. I thank her for sharing her pain, suffering, uncertainty and eventual triumph; for being vulnerable and giving us all a glimpse into her journey.

These and all the wonderful women in this book mean everything to me and I am so grateful for their participation in this book and as my friends. My world is wonderful and beautiful because of them. Thank you from the bottom of my heart, ladies.

ACKNOWLEDGMENTS

This book has been a labor of love which has come to life because of so many wonderful and amazing people. Without their generosity, grace and support, this publication would not have been possible. It took a village of many people to help me achieve my dream of becoming a transplant surgeon. I wanted to mention a few people, there are so many more I am grateful for, they fill a book on their own.

Thank you, Terrie Sizemore, my editor and publisher, visionary and writing partner, for seeing this book as a reality from that first phone call. Thank you for recognizing the importance of our voices. You have a vision for this book that was even better than the vision I have for this book. You put your soul and energy into every word and every story. Editing and reediting until it was perfect. You took time to revise and refine more than 125,000 words until it is a masterpiece. You provided critical and insightful feedback without taking away from my originality. You painstakingly fixed every error and polished this piece and now it shines! Your love and patience are invaluable.

Thank you, Brenda Carter de Treville, for copyediting, proofreading, wordsmithing, and for your insight and constructive criticism. You took time out of your busy schedule to make this dream of mine a reality. I am grateful for all the handwork you put into making this book great!

To the 74 other women who agreed to be featured in this book, thank you for believing in my vision as a place for our voices to be shared. Thank you for willing to share your stories and experiences so that others who are following behind us may benefit from them. You are ALL so inspiring and phenomenal women. I am grateful for the friendships I have developed with each and every one of you during the compiling of this book. To Mr. and Mrs. Gordon, thank you for sharing a little piece of

Sherilyn with me. I am so glad to know you.

Dr. Barbra Ross-Lee, thank you for reading every word of the book and for your insight and constructive criticism in how to make the book flow better without losing the reader. Thank you for supporting me with this book. When I was a medical student at Michigan State University College of Osteopathic Medicine, I often stood in the hallway in Fee Hall and gazed at your photo on the wall among a sea of white men. You were a trail blazer and you showed me that anything I dreamt was possible. You overcame barriers during a time when African American women physicians were not common. You went through medical school as a single mother of two children and I was motivated also as a single mother of two to succeed. You worked hard and shattered glass ceilings time and again, becoming the first black female dean of a medical school. A pioneer and legend. Thank you for showing me and others what is possible!

I am indebted to the following individuals who agreed to review the manuscript and write blurbs for me despite their own impossibly busy schedules.
- Dr. Pringl Miller
- Dr. Roberta Gebhard
- Dr. Ainhoa Costas
- Dr. Felicitas Koller
- Dr. Wendy Grant

To my wonderful and amazing work family within the surgery department at the University of Mississippi Medical Center: Dr. Christopher Anderson, Dr. Mark Earl, Dr. James Wynn, Dr. Shannon Orr, and my work sister and BFF Dr. Felicitas Koller. I am so grateful for being part of this family. I know that God brought me here for a reason and I am grateful for the support and growth during this first year of my attending life. You all have guided me and have been patient and made it a smooth transition from trainee to attending.

    I need to acknowledge a few surgeons who have made the greatest impact in my training. I am grateful to each of you that has had a hand in my development as a physician and surgeon beginning in medical school. Dr. Shirley Harding, for believing I could achieve my dream of becoming a surgeon; Dr. Susan Seman for being an example of a phenomenal clinician and surgeon early on in my training; Dr. Sample for being a great mentor to me throughout my residency, for believing in my abilities; Dr. Satterfield for being gracious to me and allowing me to have a safe place to voice my concerns when I felt I was not seen or heard; Dr. Armando Castro, for giving me a chance, without you my career would have turned out very differently; Dr. Tiszenkel, during the difficult days when I doubted and wondered if I was good enough, I went back to the words you spoke upon me as a brand new intern doing an inguinal hernia with you. You said to me, "Doctor, there are very few people I have come across in all my more than 25 years as a surgeon who have what you have; you are destined for greatness!" To this day I don't know if this is something you told every intern, but this was exactly what I needed to know that I belonged – to work hard, and excel. Ms. Donna DeChirico, thank you for your dedication to the surgeons who pass through your doors. I am grateful for all you did for me.

    To my transplant surgery family, I am grateful for all the surgeons who took the time to teach me to be a transplant surgeon. Your patience, guidance, and support throughout my two years at Nebraska Medicine is what made the long days' worth it. To my transplant father, Dr. Alan Langnas, thank you for being a great teacher, not only of the art of surgery, but also of how to talk to patients. Dr. Wendy Grant, you believed in me from the first time I met you and because of you, I am. I hear your voice the most when operating. Thank you for always being there to support me and to mold me and direct me. For all the coaching and counseling, not only for me but also for my dear transplant surgery best girlfriends, I am so grateful. I love you very much and my life is better for knowing you! Dr. Shaheed Merani, you taught me so much my first few months of fellowship; you made my transition smooth and almost easy. Thank you for taking the time to coach me a day before my general surgery boards and preparing me for the exam. Dr. Blaire Anderson, I don't have words to describe what you mean to me. Thank you for being the best litter mate. You made fellowship enjoyable. Dr. Alexander Maskin, Dr. Luciano Vargas and Dr. David Mercer, thank you for educating me and molding me into a well-rounded surgeon.

To my patients – each and every one of you that I have served and will serve – thank you for entrusting me with your care. Because of you, we are able to fulfill our life purposes of relieving pain and suffering. To the medical students, interns and residents I have worked with and work with who have taught me invaluable lessons about medicine and life, thank you.

Thank you, Sonal Johal, for helping me identify women who could contribute to the project and helping me with transcription of two of the most difficult interviews.

To my father, my late mother and my sister, Faith, I am one lucky girl to be part of this family. I appreciate your love and support through everything. Dad, thank you for reading through the first draft and for your constructive criticism. To my stepmother, I am grateful for your encouragement and input. My husband, Ryan Tiemeyer, thank you for letting me be me and for spoiling me every single day. My Shantelle and Noel, you have been through so much with me and are my constant companions and supporters. Jacob, Trent, and Daniel, Tatenda, Branden, Tiwirai, Habakuk and Hope, I am blessed to be in your lives. You all bring me so much joy. Mufaro, you light up my life. I am grateful to have a best friend like you. Shorai Ndoro-Maswela and family, I am grateful for you. Pat Burnham, Mrs. Tsikirai, Ms. Chandra, and Mama Paulina Abbey, thank you for being my prayer warriors. Dr. Shannon Davis, I appreciate you!